Yoga Through the Ages

A Distillation of Major Texts of the Yoga Traditions

Matthew Andrews

© Mathew Andrews
matthew@shraddhayoga.org

Tittle : Yoga Through the Ages

ISBN 978-93-95460-54-5 (eBook)
ISBN 978-93-95460-57-6 (Print)

BISAC Code:
HEA025000   HEALTH & FITNESS / Yoga
HEA055000   HEALTH & FITNESS / Mental Health
OCC012000   Body Mind & Spirit/Mysticism
OCC015000 Body Mind & Spirit/New Thought

Thema Subject Category:
QDHC2, Yoga (as a philosophy)
VFMG1, Yoga for exercise
VXA   Mind, body, spirit: thought and practice
VXM, Mind, body, spirit: meditation and visualization
V Health, Relationships and Personal development

Cataloging-in-Publication Data for this title is available from the Library of Congress.

Published by:
PRISMA, an imprint of Digital Media Initiatives
PRISMA, Aurelec/ Prayogshala,
Auroville 605101, Tamil Nadu, India
www.prisma.haus

Introduction

I first visited India in 2000 as part of a university study abroad program. It was September, the end of summer before the monsoon, and it was hot. Jet-lagged and hungry, I emerged into the muggy Chennai night with a sense of exhilaration. It was my twenty-first birthday, and I had finally come home.

The sense of being at home in India was not based on any outer experience. The sights, sounds and smells were new, exotic. I didn't understand the language; the food was strange and spicy; and I recoiled in the face of poverty and filth. But my soul felt a sense of relief and comfort that's like what you might feel after returning home after a long journey. I felt all of these things at the same time, and somehow there was no contradiction. The combination felt entirely natural.

I arrived in Auroville, a fascinating experiment in community that was given birth by a woman known as The Mother. She was the spiritual collaborator of the famous Indian revolutionary-turned-yogi Sri Aurobindo, and reverence for both of them was evident in their ubiquitous photographs and volumes of books. My sense of being at home resonated not just with India as a place but with Auroville, Mother, and Sri Aurobindo specifically. During the few months that I spent there in the fall of 2000 this feeling of connection strengthened and solidified within me. I knew that my future was connected to their work.

I assumed when I left Auroville and India in December that I would go right back. It was so clear to me that my path led there. But instead I was taken on a thirteen-year journey that included meeting my guru, starting a family, and working in senior leadership for an international NGO. Through all that time I would often awake in the night from a dream about Auroville with an ache in my heart. My dreams would bring me there in a very tangible way: I could see the bright auburn earth and vibrant green forest, smell the burning garbage and incense, feel the mix of dust and sweat on my skin, and sense the comfort of home in my soul.

In 2013 I was in a deep meditation, crying out to the Divine for direction, and the form of The Mother appeared in front of me. "Go to India, to Auroville," she said. "NOW." The call was so strong, so visceral and vibrant that within two weeks my wife Corinne and I were on a plane headed for Chennai. The decision to listen to this call has shaped the subsequent trajectory of my life in unbelievable ways. This writing seeks to share some of what I have experienced during that journey.

During the thirteen years between my trips to India, my reverence, awe, and devotion to my guru, whose name is Guruji-Ma (http://www.lightomega.org/), all deepened and expanded. She taught me about love, integrity, and standing for truth. She taught me discernment and the difference between having spiritual ideas and embodying them. This practical and deeply personal spiritual training was joined with my ongoing reading and exploration of the teachings of Sri Aurobindo and The Mother. The collection of essays that you are reading emerges from that joining. It is an attempt to articulate my understanding of yoga that has been fostered through deep, consistent immersion in the streams of wisdom coming from these two sources, fused with my study of many texts from the yoga tradition and fascination with the Sanskrit language.

One thing that I've noticed in my study of yogic texts is that engaging with them means engaging with layers of meaning. There are the texts themselves: ancient, written in Sanskrit or Tamil or other derivative languages, relating the experiences of the authors who lived within a particular historical milieu and had unique spiritual experiences. Then there are the commentaries and interpretations of others who have studied the texts. There is a rich tradition of commentaries in India, rooted in an approach to philosophy that's similar to the aspirations of modern physics: they were seeking a Theory of Everything. So texts were analyzed and dissected and ground to a powder to ensure that they accounted for every possible phenomena, experience, and observable situation that could arise in life. The main difference from modern physics is that there was no dogma of materialism: supra-physical phenomena like the power to see the future or be in two places at once or move objects with the mind were often accepted, and thus had to be integrated into the theory.

Yoga is an infinitely complex landscape of intersecting lineages, traditions, and streams of wisdom. Sometimes these streams crash into each other and create a swirl of conflicting ideas and stories. Sometimes they merge sweetly and harmoniously. What I have written inherently oversimplifies these interactions and relationships, the arguments and collaborations that have taken place over thousands of years. And inevitably I assert my own feelings, ideas and perspectives. In this way I join a long line of commentators who have interpreted and contextualized the writings of yoga for thousands of years and who shared the texts through the prism of their own inner experience.

I am not a technical scholar. My understanding of Sanskrit is limited, and I have a skeptical view of all the historical theories I have come across related to the origins of yoga. What I draw from most is years of seeking the place where spirit and matter mingle. I've attempted to write something that shares more than just information about the history of yoga, something that is relevant to a modern western life. These ancient texts carry a depth of practical wisdom that offers us new ways of understanding our present milieu. I've tried to bring some of that wisdom into expression.

Chronology

I've chosen to write about a specific group of texts with which I am most familiar. These texts contain different perspectives and approaches and voices, but they all align with the stream of practical wisdom that is yoga. I have presented them in a rough order based partly on historical sequence and partly on my feeling that they build upon each other. The below timeline reflects my basic sense of the timing of their development, and I've included it because many people have requested it. But not only am I unqualified to deconstruct the various arguments attempting to date these texts, I really don't find much value in the effort. I agree with the traditional perspective that the original foundational texts of yoga were received from "higher realms" than our own, and that they exist outside the bounds of time and space. I believe that they are themselves eternal, and that they flow from an eternal source.

Below is a table that lists the texts mentioned in this book and what the yoga tradition and modern scholars have to say about when they were written. The table is not a statement of truth but a general reference to help you get a sense of how the texts seem to have flowed sequentially and how the flow of wisdom may have emerged over time.

Text	According to Yoga Tradition	According to Modern Scholars
Rig Veda	conceived in the mind of God before Time was created	composed between 4000 and 1500 BCE
Upanishads	conceived in the mind of God before Time was created	the principle Upanishads were composed between 7th century and 0 BCE; minor Upanishads have been composed throughout the past two millennia
Rāmāyana	composed at the end of the Treta Yuga over 800,000 years ago	composed between the 7th and 4th centuries BCE
Bhagavad Gītā	composed at the end of the Dvarupa Yuga – around 3000 BCE	composed between 1500 and 800 BCE
Yoga Sūtras	composed by the sage Patañjali, who was an incarnation of Anantashesha, Vishnu's 7-headed serpent	compiled between 500 BCE and 300 CE by one or many yogis or possibly Buddhists
Devīmāhātmya	a story told in the future by the sage Markandeya, reflecting on events that have not yet happened	added to the Markandeya Purāna during the 5th/6th centuries

Purāṇas	often assumed to have been spoken by divine beings either to humans or other divine beings throughout the ages	wide ranging dates of composition – from the first few centuries BCE to the 16th century
Tirumantirām	compiled by devotees of a yogi who possessed the body of a dead cowherd named Mulan and spoke only one verse per year for 3,000 years	written in 200 BCE by Thirumular
Tantrasāra	written by Abhinavagupta around 1000 CE	written by Abhinavagupta around 1000 CE
Ramacharitamanasa	written by Tulasidasa - a reincarnation of Valmiki - in the 16th century CE	written by Tulasidasa in the 16th century CE
Savitrī	written by Sri Aurobindo between 1910 and 1950 CE	written by Sri Aurobindo between 1910 and 1950 CE

In our modern world the word 'science' has taken on the flavor that was invested in 'Christianity' in medieval Europe. Science has become like a religion with fundamental materialism as its dogma, and this shapes our common understanding of history. The reality is that there is still more that we don't know or can't explain than what we can, and a humble approach to the history of yoga takes the texts at face value rather than imposing our materialist dogma on them. Humility leaves room for mysticism, magic and divine intervention in human affairs, and lets us stay open to receiving what the texts have to offer.

I am making a distinction here between 'science' as the word has come into common parlance, and the scientific method, which is directly linked to the science of yoga. The scientific method invites us to investigate our own experience, whether in waking life, in our dreams and imagination, or in the depths of silent meditation. We find what is real by investigating and comparing our experiences over time, referencing the experiences of others as related in ancient texts and modern videos, and always seeking the embodied sense of truth that exceeds the mind's fragmented and distorted understandings. The scientific method when separated from the dogma of materialism and applied to our subjective experience, the deepening experience of the source of our conscious awareness, is the essence of yoga practice.

The modern capitalist yoga culture manipulates the mystique of yoga to engage consumers and sell products. Many modern yoga teachers and businesses, some with a superficial understanding of yoga and no expression of honor or gratitude to the Indian culture that produced it, have used the aura of an ancient mystical science that promises liberation from suffering to profit themselves at the expense of others. So while maintaining humility and reverence for the teachings themselves, we can leverage the deepening of discernment that yoga offers to thread the needle between the hubris of modern 'science' and the rampant cultural appropriation of modern yoga culture.

This includes your engagement with this book, dear reader. I have spent decades studying yoga and traveling back and forth from India, compelled by a love for yoga that even I don't fully understand. All I can offer you is my own lens, my own heart, my learnings and perspectives. This book is an offering at the feet of Ādiyogeshvara, the Lord of Yoga. I pray that it serve the purposes of awakening and freedom from suffering that yoga has served for thousands of years, and I ask that you forgive the places where my ego asserts itself and obscures the truth.

Some Notes on Sanskrit and Translations

Every translation that you ever read of anything anywhere has a major element of subjectivity to it. This is particularly true of Sanskrit to English translations because the voice of the languages is so different. Sanskrit is packed, dense, with no prepositions, and some textual formats (sūtras for example) extend that by often leaving out verbs as well. To translate directly into English would render the text terse, dry and flat. Beyond that there are often many possible word-to-word translations from Sanskrit to English, so choosing the right word in the right context adds a whole additional layer of challenge. Every translator makes choices about how much to emphasize poetics, whether to align with a particular philosophy, how to treat different grammatical elements, and how to capture the author's voice and intent. Every translation is a product of those choices. This is just as true for me as it is for anyone else. Unless otherwise noted the translations in this book are my own, using my fairly basic understanding of Sanskrit grammar and vocabulary, and often using several other translations as inspiration.

To me the best way to engage with a text like the Yoga Sūtra or the Bhagavad Gītā is to read many different translations, especially ones that provide a breakdown of the Sanskrit words and grammar, and then feel for yourself what seems to convey truth. Part of this feeling comes through the words themselves; more than any modern language, the sounds of Sanskrit words sonically convey their meaning. By saying them aloud, listening to them, chanting them, and exploring them, an embodied sense of the words tends to arise without needing to figure it out with the mind. This way of engaging directly with the phrases and the words that form them offers us a path through the dense thicket of divergent and contradictory interpretations and commentaries that have been offered by countless pundits throughout the ages.

I've chosen to italicize Sanskrit words throughout this book to highlight and differentiate them. I've also used a specific transliteration scheme. Because Sanskrit and English have different alphabets, there are letters that appear in Sanskrit that do not have a direct English equivalent. And because Sanskrit is a phonetic language, the only way to understand how to pronounce a word is to have the exact spelling. Some Sanskrit letters are easy enough to transfer into English; for example, there are letters in Sanskrit that represent long vowels and short vowels. So while we can say the letter a several different ways – can, want, late, fast, etc – in Sanskrit a is always pronounced like the u in but. And there's another symbol that is always pronounced like the a in water. In this book, I've transcribed the short a as a, and the long a as ā.

But there are some symbols that are not so simple to render into English. There is a standard Sanskrit transliteration scheme called the IAST, but it includes symbols that are not easy for me to replicate on my MacBook keyboard, so I've chosen to leave those out. This omission honestly pains me, but I'm just not up to the painstaking task of hunting and pecking every glottal nasal and palatal stop. In Sanskrit there are four symbols for our *n*, three for our *t* and *d*, and a symbol that indicates a nasalization of the preceding vowel, basing the choice of nasal on the subsequent consonant. So I've indicated long and short vowels, but that's all. In other cases I've written the word as closely to how it should sound as I reasonably can. Please forgive me.

Pronunciation Scheme

a is pronounced like but
ā is pronounced like father
ai is like aisle
au is like cow

i is like bit
ī is like sweet
u is like put
ū is like flute
e is always like lay
o is always like goat
c is always like cheese, never like license
ch is like church-house
dh is like madhouse
th is like hothouse
ph is always like uphill, never like elephant
gh is always like doghouse, never like through or trough
jh is like sledgehammer
kh is like backhoe
n may be north or sing or turn, depending on what it would normally be in English
ñ is like onion
ś is like shoesh is like shun
v is somewhere between vet and wet
y is always like yes and never like hilly.

Two Special Characters – Visarga and Anusvara

Generally, when h is at the end of a word or in a place that it seems like it shouldn't be (like the first h in duhkha), it adds a slight breath to the preceding vowel; at the end of a sentence it also adds a slight echo to the preceding vowel. This breath/echo and the symbol that represents it are called the *visarga*.

There is a special character in Sanskrit called the *anusvara*, which indicates a nasalization of the preceding vowel, basing the choice of nasal on the subsequent consonant. Simple right? So in the word *Sanskrit* for example, the *n* is not actually an *n*. It's an *anusvara*. The reason we pronounce it as an *n* is that the next letter is *skri*, and the nasal that corresponds to *skri* is *n*. If the next letter was *pa*, like in *sampatti*, then the *anusvara* would be pronounced as an *m*. The way I've represented the *anusvara* in this book is that I've written the English letter that it sounds like when the word is pronounced. When it shows up at the end of a word, then I just used *m*, and I'll trust you to remember that the pronunciation will change depending on the first consonant of the next word in the *mantra*, *rik*, *sūtra*, or phrase. Just to add a little more spice to the curry, the way *anusvara* is transliterated in the IAST is the symbol *ṃ*. So if we use the IAST, it looks like it's supposed to be pronounced as an *ṃ*. Is this deep enough into the weeds for you?

Contents

Introduction

Chapter 1   The Rig Veda and the Roots of Yoga   1

Chapter 2   The Rig Veda – Evolution, Light and Darkness   13

Chapter 3   The Upanishads – Inner Reality   23

Chapter 4   The Rāmāyana – Bhakti, Dhārma, and Karma   39

Chapter 5   Sankhya Kārikā – Enumerating Reality   53

Chapter 6   Patañjali's Yoga Sūtra – The Path of Purification   75

Chapter 7   Bhagavad Gītā – The Great Synthesis   101

Chapter 8   The Devīmāhātmya – Glory of the Divine Mother   119

Chapter 9   Thirumanthiram and Tantrāloka – Gifts of Śiva   137

Chapter 10 Savitri – A Legend And A Symbol   159

Bibliography   179

Chapter - 1

The Rig Veda and the Roots of Yoga

yo jāgāra tam ṛcaḥ kāmayante
"The one who is awake, the hymns (of the Veda) seek him out."

Rig Veda 5.44.14

What is Yoga? It's a word and idea that has flowed into and saturated popular culture in the United States. Mention the word to a stranger at the supermarket or the bank, and you will likely meet with a basic understanding and familiarity. And while we know that yoga arises from an ancient tradition with roots in India, what most modern westerners think of when they hear the word *yoga* is something entirely new, a modern creation. This modern creation surely has value, but it is quite different from how yoga has been understood in India for thousands of years.

When people say *yoga* in the modern United States, the association is most often to some form of asana or posture practice. Asana is a small aspect of the vast scope of yoga, which encompasses every area of life. While most yoga teacher trainings in the west use *Patanjali's Yoga Sūtras* as their primary reference text, most Indians have never heard of this book (although as western yoga flows from west to east, the *Yoga Sūtras* are becoming more widely known in India), and they surely haven't read it. But they have heard of the *Vedas*, the

Upanishads, the *Rāmāyana*, the *Mahābhārata*, the *Devī Bhāgavatam*, and the *Śiva Purāna*. These works have not only been read and memorized and shared within families and communities for millennia, they have inspired countless temples, sculptures, paintings, songs, poems, dramas, and dances. So if we seek to truly understand and honor yoga, we must go beneath the surface of what our modern culture has created and seek something deeper.

And the depth of yoga obviously speaks to some inner need in our modern culture. People could choose to go to any kind of fitness class, but for some reason they choose yoga. The deep spiritual resonance calls to them, inviting them to explore aspects of themselves that hunger to be seen and honored. And the more we, as yoga teachers, can understand and share from that depth, the more directly we respond to that often inarticulate hunger.

So let's start at the beginning, or at least as close to the beginning as we can get. We can't really understand yoga without understanding the *Rig Veda*. The four *Vedas* (*Rig Veda*, *Sāma Veda*, *Yajur Veda*, *Atharva Veda*) are the foundation of yoga, and the *Rig Veda* is the first of the four. In fact the additional three, while they do contain a great deal of new material, also restate, recontextualize, and explain how to engage the hymns of the *Rig Veda*. No one knows for sure when these texts were written down and how long they had been transmitted orally before that. Within the broader yoga tradition they are generally considered to be timeless, existing outside of the duality of time and space, spoken by the Divine Oneness before the Earth was born, and passed on to humanity verbatim. They are considered a living being, embodied as *Gāyatrī*, an aspect of the Divine Mother.

The Vedic corpus, which includes the *Upanishads*, are distinguished as śruti or heard, as opposed to the other *smriti* or conceived texts in the yogic tradition. They were not authored by the Vedic rishis who composed them but received via transmission from the One, an act of establishing connection with humanity.

> ṛco akṣare paramé vyoman
> yasmin devā adhi viśve niṣeduḥ
> yas tan na veda kim ṛcā kariṣyati
> ya it tad vidus ta ime samāsate

The imperishable hymns (of the Veda) rest in the place beyond all space, in which reside the devās (the radiant ones), the primal forces that manifest the universe.
Whoever does not know (or is not open to) this place, what will the hymns accomplish for them? Those who do know this place find perfect stability (balance, evenness).

Rig Veda 1.164.39

The problem is that the *Rig Veda* is not at all easy to understand. When western anthropologists first encountered it they concluded that it was a bunch of animistic songs worshipping various natural phenomena (the sun, the rain, fire, water, etc.) and regaling tribal feuds. Even among Indian scholars there has been little agreement about a coherent and consistent message to be derived from the *Vedas*. The rituals that are woven throughout what is currently called Hinduism include *Vedic* mantras, prayers and practices, but they have often been reduced to superstitious appeals for personal/familial material gain. The stories and characters that populate the *Vedas* are told individually, but without an underlying sense of a unified message or narrative.

The strange thing about all this is that the most profound and beautiful yogic texts, including the *Upanishads*, the *Mahābhārata* and the *Bhagavad Gītā*, the *Rāmāyana*, and the many *Purānas*, refer directly to the *Vedas* as fundamental, true, and vitally important.

These subsequent texts that rest upon the Vedas as a foundation are deeply insightful about individual and collective human psychology, and quite advanced philosophically. So what's missing?

> *"The Veda is a book of esoteric symbols, almost of spiritual formulae, which masks itself as a collection of ritual poems."*
> The Secret of the Veda by Sri Aurobindo p.233

If you look at most English translations of the *Rig Veda*, it does indeed appear to be a collection of hymns to deities that represent aspects of nature – *Agni* the fire, *Sūrya* the sun, *Usha* the dawn, *Sarasvatī* the river, *Varuna* the ocean, *Indra* the thunderbolt, *Rudra* the howling storm. And one of the central themes of the *Rig Veda* involves Indra vanquishing the *Vritra* and the *panis*, enemies that had stolen the āryans' cows and hidden them in a cave. The hymns are beautiful and worthy of admiration. But it's hard to see how tribal animistic hymns would be considered fundamental to the profound wisdom of the *Upanishads*.

The "Secret" Double Meaning of the Veda

Sri Aurobindo, the great Indian scholar, revolutionary, poet and yogi, introduced a new and fascinating idea about these ancient mysterious works. He was a linguistic genius who deeply understood the roots of many of the Indo-European languages and used this understanding to open a door to a new understanding of Vedic Sanskrit, and the *Vedas* themselves. He says that the *Vedas* contain a hidden double meaning that underlies the surface concepts. For example, he equates *Agni* not just with material fire, but with the fire of aspiration, the fire of the soul's desire to exceed, grow in capacity, manifest increasingly within the life of an individual. He says that when the *rishis* sing to *Agni*, they are praising and calling out to the embodiment of this quality, asking it to infuse them.

> "Agni is a god – He is of the Devas, the shining ones, the Master of the light – the great cosmic gamesters, the lesser lords of the Lila, of which Yajña is the Maheshwara, our Almighty Lord. He is fire and unbound or binds himself only in play. He is inherently pure, and he is not touched or soiled by the impurity on which he feeds. He enjoys the play of good and evil and leads, raises, or forces the evil towards goodness. He burns in order to purify. He destroys in order to save. When the body of the Sadhaka is burned up with the heat of the Tapas, it is Agni that is roaring and devouring and burning up in him the impurity and the obstructions. He is a dreadful, mighty, blissful, merciless and loving God, the kind and fierce helper of all who take refuge in his friendship."
>
> Hymns to the Mystic Fire by Sri Aurobindo pp.439-40

Sri Aurobindo equates *Saraswatī* not just with a river, but with divine inspiration that flows from above and pours into the human consciousness, offering insights and possibilities that exceed the limited mentality. He equates *Indra* not just with the thunderbolt, but with the illumined mind, awareness awakened to its own divine origins. And these connections are not just metaphor: these beings are embodiments of the qualities that they represent, as well as personifications that manifest as natural phenomena. When we see a flame, we see *Agni* there, burning and reaching toward heaven.

> "The Gods are not simply poetical personifications of abstract ideas or of psychological and physical functions of Nature. To the Vedic seers they are living realities; the vicissitudes of the human soul represent a cosmic struggle not merely of principles and tendencies but of the cosmic Powers which support and embody them. These are the Gods and the Demons. On the world-stage and in the individual soul the same real drama with the same personages is enacted."
>
> Hymns to the Mystic Fire by Sri Aurobindo p.30

> *"Who is this Yajña and what is this Agni? Yajña, the Master of the Universe, is the universal living Intelligence who possesses and controls His world; Yajña is God. Agni also is a living intelligence that has gone forth from the Personality to do His work and represent His power; Agni is a god. The material sense sees neither God nor gods, neither Yajña nor Agni; it sees only the elements and the formations of the elements, material appearances and the movements in or of those appearances. It does not see Agni, it sees a fire; it does not see God, it sees the earth green and the sun flaming in heaven and is aware of the wind that blows and the waters that roll. So too it sees the body or appearance of a man, not the man himself; it sees the look or the gesture, but of the thought behind the look or gesture it is not aware. Yet the man exists in the body and thought exists in the look or gesture. So too Agni exists in the fire and God exists in the world."*
>
> Hymns to the Mystic Fire by Sri Aurobindo pp.439-40

This double meaning also extends to the sacrificial rituals that arise from, and are woven throughout the *Vedas*. The sacrifice, or *yajña*, includes lighting the fire, offering ghee and *soma*, and chanting sacred mantras. The symbolism is both psychological and spiritual. The ghee represents the light of the awakened mind. When offered to the fire, the flames of aspiration digest the offering and surge toward heaven, releasing the subtlest aspect of the offering as smoke and leaving the denser aspect behind as pure ash. The flame purifies the offering of our illumined intelligence and delivers it to the Divine. The *soma* is the secret joy of being that hides within all sensation, all life force, and thus flows through the stem and vine of every living plant. The *devas*, or radiant ones, helpers of humanity, are invited to come and share the drink and by it they are fortified and their strength increases. And the sacred word also both attracts the divine helpers and expands their strength. We call upon beings of light to support our quest for spiritual growth, and they fly to us like bees to flowers, nourished by our call.

> "The sacrifice is the giving by man of what he possesses in his being to the higher or divine nature, and its fruit is the farther enrichment of his manhood by the lavish bounty of the gods.... the sacrifice is a journey, a progression; the sacrifice itself travels led by Agni up the divine path to the gods...[and it is] also a battle, for it is opposed by the Panis, Vritras, and other powers of evil and falsehood."
>
> The Secret of the Veda by Sri Aurobindo p.234

One of the central legends of the *Rig Veda*, which weaves itself throughout, is the story of the *Angirasa rishis* who rescue the Sun and its rays out of the dark cave where it was hidden by the *panis* – undivine beings who do no sacrifice, hate the divine word, and gather wealth that they can't use because they don't know how. The *panis* are powers of darkness that oppose the spiritual seeker, and the devas are the powers of light and truth that give support. It happens that the word *go* in Sanskrit can mean both cow and light. If it is taken to mean *cow*, then the whole legend can be reduced to a human battle between a tribal enemy who has stolen the Aryans' cows and hidden them in a cave. But if *go* is taken to mean *light*, then the whole sense of the legend changes and we have a story about the light of truth being hidden by forces of darkness, and then freed by the devas.

> "If Vritra and the waters symbolize the cloud and the rain and the gushing forth of the seven rivers of the Punjab and if the Angirasas are the bringers of the physical dawn, then the Veda is a symbolism of natural phenomena personified in the figure of gods and Rishis and maleficent demons. If Vritra and Vala are Dravidian gods and the Panis and Vritras human enemies, then the Veda is a poetical and legendary account

> of the invasion of Dravidian India by Nature-worshipping barbarians. If on the other hand this is a symbolism of the struggle between spiritual powers of Light and Darkness, Truth and Falsehood, Knowledge and Ignorance, Death and Immortality, then that is the real sense of the whole Veda."
>
> The Secret of the Veda by Sri Aurobindo p.233

Collective Spiritual Evolution

In the modern west, we credit Darwin with "discovering" evolution. But millennia before Darwin, the *Vedas* describe a process of evolution through which life evolves from matter, and mind evolves from life. This evolution is preceded by an involution, through which mind and life embed themselves within matter, setting the stage for them to emerge through time. The Divine One secreted Themself within the dense ignorance of matter and then began a process of unveiling through the gradual and intricate processes of Nature. Life emerged from matter: self-regulating and expanding. Then mind emerged from life, with even more capacity for unifying and synthesizing.

And the *Vedas* tell us that beyond mind is further growth, the evolution of a wisdom that harmonizes opposites, synthesizes truth, experiences the underlying unity of the cosmos. We sit today at the edge of the mind's ability to lead us into the future, and a collective call is arising within human hearts for a new capacity that exceeds the mind's limitations. The *Vedas* tell us that this new capacity will change everything: even matter itself will be transformed and divinized as we open to the future. What comes is as radical as the change from plant to fish, or from fish to mammal, or from mammal to human being.

Sri Aurobindo's revelation is profound, nuanced, and multi-faceted. Even he acknowledged that the two major books he wrote about the

Vedas (*The Secret of the Veda* and *Hymns to the Mystic Fire*) just begin to scratch the surface and offer a glimpse of their significance. His work has many implications for teaching yoga in the modern west.

First, the *Vedas* are the roots of yoga. Everything that comes after comes from this source. And the *Vedas* declare that everything is holy – every life, every breath, every fall, every death is part of the vast collective sweep of God's revelation and manifestation. They are hymns of praise to real beings of love that are born from and serve the Oneness and Unity that underlie all existence. The natural world and our inner world are one world, a world that grows increasingly toward wholeness with help from the One divine being in all Its various manifestations. These divine beings/forces influence our daily life, drawing us along the path of self-realization that is the same path that the whole Earth travels. We sing to these beings and offer praise and gratitude to them in order to empower them and increase their support of our spiritual growth.

But there are also forces that seek to arrest this growth, forces that seek to increase our sense of separation, isolation, and confusion. The *Vedas* describe a world that is evolving out of darkness and into light, out of ignorance and into knowledge. The advance of light and truth is opposed by forces of darkness and ignorance, but light is stronger and always prevails, not by destroying the darkness but just by being, and by growing stronger in its own radiance. The *Vedas* tell us that, in an ancient and Divine collaboration, truth seeks to manifest on Earth and the Earth seeks to manifest truth – the realms of matter and spirit need not be and will not be forever separate.

> *"The antinomy between the Light and the Darkness, the Truth and the Falsehood, has its roots in an original cosmic antinomy between the illumined Infinite and the darkened finite consciousness. Aditi, the infinite, the undivided is the*

mother of the Gods; Diti or Danu, the division, the separative consciousness is the mother of the Titans. Therefore the gods in us move towards light, infinity, and unity; the titans dwell in their cave of the darkness and issue from it only to break up, make discordant, wounded, limited our knowledge, will, strength, joy, and being."

The Secret of the Veda by Sri Aurobindo p.421

Cosmic Forces in Everyday Life

What has come to be known as yoga is rooted in an ancient spiritual tradition that, in a very nuanced and specific way, describes a world that is much more complex and multidimensional than we typically assume. The *Rig Veda* points to cosmic forces that interpenetrate our individual lives – influencing our thoughts, feelings, and beliefs. We are not the isolated beings that we thought we were, enclosed in our skin. Energies, forces of light and darkness, forces that support our growth toward wholeness and forces that seek to block that growth, forces of love and forces of separation move through us, under the radar, but with real effect. Every event in our individual and collective lives can be understood differently through this lens. Our lives take on an inherent sense of purpose, something that many in our modern world are lacking and hungering for.

People today are spiritually starving. They long for connection, for hope, for the experience of being seen and being loved. The *Vedas* tell us that this hunger, this aspiration, is natural. It is not to be ignored or suppressed, but kindled, empowered and sung out. Our longing for wholeness is as natural as fire, and it purifies us; it burns away separation. It reaches toward heaven and releases an offering of smoke; it lights up the darkness, and it offers warmth and protection. Nurturing our aspiration draws collaborative forces of light to us, empowers them, and transforms life from a chaotic dog-eat-dog scramble to a purposeful adventure of self-discovery.

The ancient teachings of yoga call to us and invite us to understand ourselves and the world around us more deeply, to pay attention and take notice. The major problems that we face today: personally, locally, nationally, and globally, look insoluble to the separative mechanistic consciousness. But the more we understand the hidden forces that are at play, how they operate and what motivates them, the more possibilities emerge for approaching problems from the inside, by dealing directly with fundamental energies. Then teaching yoga becomes an opportunity to hold a deeper perspective on life and offer it to those who are drawn to you as a guide and friend.

> *"The Rig Veda rises out of the ancient Dawn with the sound of a thousand-voiced hymn lifted from the soul of [humanity] to an all-creative Truth and an all-illumining Light. Truth and Light are synonymous or equivalent words in the thought of the Vedic seers even as are their opposites, Darkness and Ignorance. The battle of the Vedic Gods and Titans is a perpetual conflict between Day and Night for the possession of the triple world of heaven, mid-air, and earth and for the liberation or bondage of the mind, life and body of the human being, his mortality or his immortality. It is waged by the Powers of a supreme Truth and Lords of a supreme Light against other dark Powers who struggle to maintain the foundation of this falsehood in which we dwell and the iron walls of these hundred fortified cities of the Ignorance."*
>
> The Secret of the Veda by Sri Aurobindo p.421

Chapter - 2

The Rig Veda – Evolution, Light and Darkness

Yoga is life seeking to expand, to exceed itself. Yoga is the emergent future, the rising sun, the persistent evolutionary movement: from the rock to the plant to the fish, amphibian, reptile, bird, mammal, ape, human…and? Refining and assimilating and attempting, testing an endless variety of possibilities, but always expanding, widening.

Life's emergence from matter was nothing short of miraculous. However it may have happened, a self-organizing, self-individuating, self-preserving tendency developed in the Earth's primordial waters. Bacteria bloomed and joined to create multi-cellular organisms, algae, plankton. Life diversified and expanded, climbing out of the water and fixing itself on land, flowering and flourishing. And as life individuated further, the self-organizing capacity expanded into fish, amphibians, reptiles and mammals, individual untethered beings with proto-brains and proto-egos.

Evolution continued and mind coalesced into a container for consciousness. Mind allows the experience of self as an individual to reach an entirely new level. Mind looks around and sees *not-self* and differentiates that from self. Mind allows the ego, the container of self-identity, to define, refine, and set like a jelly mold. And mind too grows and expands, faster even than life, because now it can grow without killing. Two minds join and build on each other, expanding exponentially. Before writing, the growth of mind was limited by memory and death, but writing extended learning eternally into the future. Before intercontinental travel, mind was limited by perspective and subject to the perimeters of cultural norms, but now the internet has opened the doors to exponential noetic expansion.

Mind has its own limitations. It cannot easily reconcile conflicting ideas; it cannot see wholes, only pieces. It cannot know another being from the inside, only from the outside. And for this reason, it cannot solve any of the critical global social problems that we face today. What can overcome these limitations? What can overstep these bounds?

Every day we take for granted miracles that could not have been fathomed or believed just 200 years ago, not to mention 2,000 or 2,000,000 years. Consider jet planes from the perspective of anyone living in the year 1700, or bananas in New England, motion pictures, laparoscopic heart surgery, vaccines, Wikipedia, Google, or video chatting across continents for free. Our consciousness evolves as technologies shrink the world and demolish barriers to experiencing life through the eyes of the "other". We begin to tolerate differences in culture, in life experience, in belief systems, and then protect them, and then celebrate them. The future is emerging, and what is to come will be as unimaginable to our modern sensibilities as mind would have been to a bacterium or a fish or a monkey. Evolution is not over.

Yoga yokes us to the future. And the future is love. We, in general and as a whole, are becoming more open, more receptive, more caring, more collaborative than humans in the past. Of course, there are forces that push back against this movement. According to Sri Aurobindo's model for understanding, the *Rig Veda*, our universe contains a fundamental tension between forces of light and forces of darkness. Forces of light seek to support and increase truth, while forces of darkness seek to increase falsehood. These forces influence cosmic and global events, as well as the day-to-day events of our individual lives.

Forces of light support our identification and union with our essential self. Light is love and truth absolutely wedded to each other, but it's not an idea; it's a force, a substance, an energy that acts and interacts with our multi-layered selves. Light is embodied in the devas of the Veda, the beings who seek the highest good for each and for all, and who draw us ever toward the experience of being, giving, and receiving Divine Love. The devas nurture experiences of connection, safety, peace, hope and acceptance. They nourish the seeker and empower the search for Truth, reality, wholeness.

Forces of darkness oppose light, and push us toward identification with a separated, isolated ego. Darkness is embodied in the Vedic *asuras*, *panis* and *dasyus*, who stoke experiences of fear, anxiety, confusion, alienation, loneliness, and anger. The *asuras* act on collectives, influencing leaders of national and multinational entities, while the *dasyus* and *panis* act on a smaller scale, but using the same tactics and seeking the same ends. They all work through the ego's vulnerabilities and amplify its sense of separateness. And since we are mostly unconscious of the source of our thoughts, they use thought as a tool to sow confusion and doubt about our divine nature. As we begin to dis-identify with our thoughts, we can watch them move through us, infiltrating from outside, interacting with our own collection of karmic inclinations, and reinforcing the structure of beliefs that forms the ego's fortress and prison.

Sūrya: The Sun

Sūrya is a leader of the Vedic legions of light. He is the Sun, and just as with *Agni* and the other Vedic devas, *Sūrya* has a physical form that we can see and feel via our external senses, but he is also a Being that encompasses and contains more than the material. We can touch *Sūrya* with our inner senses through the emotions that the Sun evokes in us, through a range of solar symbols and metaphors, and by opening directly to his essence, or soul qualities.

Agni's qualities are heat, light, and purification. *Sūrya* shares these qualities, but they are both vaster and more distant, more radiant but less within our control. He is praised in *Rig Veda* Book 1 as "the highest Light of all," and in Book 10 as "all-seeing Intelligence," and "the far-seeing eye of knowledge." He is both illumination, the radiance through which darkness and falsehood are dispelled, and he is the seer that perceives the truth, discerning the real from the unreal, knowledge from ignorance. Sri Aurobindo calls *Sūrya* "the light of the Truth rising on the human consciousness." *Sūrya* "goes where the gods have made a path for him." The other devas support us, releasing the hold that ignorance has placed upon us. *Sūrya*, following in their wake, pours down from above the infinite light of truth.

> "*Sūrya*, the Sun, is the master of [the] supreme Truth – truth of being, truth of knowledge, truth of process and act and movement and functioning. He is therefore the creator or rather the manifester of all things, for creation is outbringing, expression by the Truth and Will, and the father, fosterer, enlightener of our souls. The illuminations we seek are the herds of this Sun who comes to us in the track of the divine Dawn and release and reveal in us night-hidden world after world up to the highest Beatitude."
>
> Hymns to the Mystic Fire by Sri Aurobindo p.31

Sūrya is also known by other names which are applied to his specific qualities. *Savitrī* is the Creator, the Awakener, the divine action of light that penetrates darkness and opens new possibilities. *Savitrī* illumines our consciousness, stirs aspiration within us, awakens us from the dream that we had mistaken for reality. *Savitrī* plants the seeds of tomorrow in today's soil and then coaxes them out of their husks, drawing their tendrils up through the crust of earth and into the open air.

> *"Om, Earth, Heaven, and the Region Between. We fix our consciousness on the glorious Savitrī, purifying radiance of the devas. Please illuminate our minds."*
>
> The Gayatri Mantra: Rig Veda Mandala III, Sukta 62, Mantra 10

Pūshan is another aspect of *Sūrya*. He is the Increaser, day-by-day fostering, nourishing, expanding our consciousness and capacity to embody truth. *Pūshan* embodies the evolutionary impulse, reaching ever higher, climbing through the ages and always increasing, expanding, widening. He is the force of purification that clears away the darkness that clings to us, flushing it out from hiding and into the light of day. *Pūshan* is our experience of Truth that grows with each new dawn and never recedes, expands ever toward the horizon, encompasses more and more of the infinite sacred wholeness that underlies everything everywhere. *Sūrya* does not just disappear into the depth of night and reappear each morning in an endless static cycle. Each dawn is new, entirely unlike any dawn that has come before, breaking ground and ushering in the future.

This tension between light and darkness exists in the universe, and it also influences both the macrocosm of geopolitical events and the microcosm of our individual lives. If we seek to understand ourselves, to discover our essential nature and embody truth in our daily lives, then we will gain a great deal from understanding the hidden forces that inform our desires, our aversions, our aspirations, and our fears. For what we typically think of as our *self* is actually an agglomeration of forces and voices, each with its own agendas and aims, jostling and wrestling each other in an effort to control our thoughts and actions. The ego itself is a veil that hides the individuality of these forces behind a gathered sense of *I, me, mine*. And as long as the essential self (*purusha*, soul, spirit, *jīvātman*, etc) remains hidden and subdued, our lives are a battlefield for these forces.

> *"A superconscient Truth lies concealed and is the basis of the infinite being which stands revealed on those higher altitudes of our ascension...[W]e have to bring forward the Truth as an offering so that the luminous god with his golden hands full of the Light may rise high in our heavens and hear our word...[W]e must widen out the cord of Savitrī so that it shall release us into higher states of life made accessible to us and harmonized within our being."*
>
> The Secret of the Veda by Sri Aurobindo p.437

The purpose of human existence, according to Sri Aurobindo, is to collaborate with the devas and forces of light, each an individualized emanation of the Divine One, in the establishment of a "Life Divine" on Earth. This divine life is the culmination of material evolution and the evolution of consciousness (which of course are not separate). And it encompasses all of life, including matter itself, which will progressively become divinized, awakened, and self-luminous. Our collective *dhārma* is to seek out the illumined ones who point the way to greater truth and yoke ourselves to them, allowing them to draw us forward into a fuller and truer version of ourselves.

> "The illumined ones yoke their minds and their thoughts to Him Who is Illumination, Largeness, and Clarity. Knowing all phenomema, He alone orders the energies of the sacrifice. Savitrī, the divine Creator, is vastly affirmed in all things."
>
> Rig Veda V.81.1

Yajña: The Vedic Sacrifice

Sri Aurobindo refutes the *Vedantic* philosophy that material reality is inherently unreal, and that the divine reality is static, unchanging. More on the nuances of that in the next chapter. Of course an eternal vastness underlies and pervades everything, but this world in which we live is born of the Divine One and thus is part of the Divine One, not separate. And it is in a process of unfoldment, of evolution.

Instead, he urges us to wake up and shake off the delusion and denial of egoism and realize the true purpose of our human lives. This purpose is the central pillar of Sri Aurobindo's Integral Yoga, and explains his claim that *All Life is Yoga*.

The conception of *yajña* or sacrifice is central to the *Vedas*. The word *sacrifice* has made its way into our modern lexicon with the insinuation of relinquishing something, letting go of something that we care about, giving something up. But sacrifice is not a loss, it is a gain. By releasing something that we have identified as *self* – whether an idea, a material object, a manner of speaking, or any other habit that calcifies around our essential self and obscures its radiance – we open ourselves to a greater experience of who we actually are.

This differentiation in self-identity is central to understanding the Vedic idea of sacrifice. For the soul, which is inherently free, eternal, and unified with all that is, embodiment as a human in the realm of duality is inherently a sacrifice. We forsake the infinite freedom, knowledge, immortality and bliss of our souls and incarnate into limitation, ignorance, death and suffering, in the process forgetting our true nature. What could be worse? Why would we choose such a thing?

The soul has chosen this self-giving willingly, and retains an understanding of why. When we shift from a self-identity as the limited and self-isolated ego to a self-identity as an immortal soul, we gain a wider perspective on the sacrifice itself. The soul gives itself willingly to life, consenting to participate in the collective evolutionary endeavor of the Earth's awakening. The Earth offers itself without reserve to every soul, and every soul offers itself to the Earth. The individual good that a separated consciousness holds so dear is released in favor of the collective good that embraces not just all of humanity, but all of life and beyond. We are not the victim of the sacrifice, but the Lord of the sacrifice, willingly offering all that we are in service of the Oneness that is God.

A Divine Life on Earth means the freeing of matter, life and mind from their inherent limitations. It means that matter will no longer decay, life will no longer feed upon death, and mind will open to a direct perception of unity. This evolutionary process has been going on and will continue whether you or I consciously participate with it or not. But the next evolutionary phase includes the collective awakening of humankind to our secret *dhārma*, our holy task, and a joining in collaboration with the forces of Light to establish love and truth on Earth.

When we harness ancient sunlight to power our modern conveniences, or derive vaccines and medicines from plants and micro-organisms, mind is shaping life and matter. Similarly, life and mind will be transformed by the influx of light that comes through this collaboration. The transformation of matter is taking place right now, in the energetic substructure of dirt, rocks, water and plants, and of course within our own bodies. This is something we can sense, feel, experience if we can release old habits of thinking and pay attention to our bodies with clear, innocent attention. Every breath offers us a doorway to direct experience of our body's cells and systems waking up to their own divinity.

Yoga is union, joining the individual with the collective, the collective with the whole, and the whole with the infinite from which it arises. The *Rig Veda* provides the context for understanding many subsequent yogic texts. Its symbology is used as a foundation and is expanded upon throughout the *Upanishads, Purānas, Rāmāyana, Mahābhārata,* and others. If we apply Sri Aurobindo's interpretation of the Veda to the dramas of these later compositions, they become practical guidebooks for navigating a purposeful life in a multi-dimensional universe.

> *"Those whose intelligence is clouded proclaim that the Vedas are all about ritualistic acts. They do not understand the Veda."*
>
> Bhagavata Purāna IV:29:8

Chapter - 3

The Upanishads – Inner Reality

In the late summer of 2002, I was wandering around at an outdoor festival in Amherst, where I had recently landed after hiking from Georgia to Connecticut on the Appalachian Trail. Alone one night in a shelter outside of Kent, Connecticut, I'd decided that waking up every day with feet exploding in pain, then walking on them until the pain faded to numbness was optional. I decided it was okay to take a break. So I took a bus to Williams, Massachusetts and hitchhiked in the direction of Amherst. The guy who picked me up was headed to a 10-day Vipassana Meditation retreat in Shelburne Falls, and I had no urgent plans so I went with him. I figured that ten days of sitting would give my feet time to heal.

A week or so after the retreat I was wandering at this festival, unsure of whether I was going back to the trail or whether I was done. I had no plans, immediate or long-term. I was maximally adrift. I stopped in at a healer's booth, and we started talking. I don't remember any of the conversation, but I remember that she asked if I ever prayed. It struck me, because I thought of myself as a serious spiritual seeker, having lived in India and at a yoga community in California, and having hiked much of the Appalachian Trail and just returned from a 10-day silent meditation retreat. I thought I was on a spiritual path. But no, actually, I didn't pray. I didn't talk to God, and I didn't listen.

That meeting stuck with me, and when I encountered the same healer at another festival a month or so later, I asked if she would teach me what she knew. She agreed, and over time she helped me to explore the inner dimensions of myself. She introduced me to the place where my individual self gives way to a cosmic Self, to the Realms of Light, and to the beings of Light who are always holding the earth with love and offering guidance to those who aspire to embody truth. She told me about her teacher and said that I could meet with her if I wanted.

I reached out to her teacher, and scheduled a time for her to call me back. I was awaiting the call at home one day, and my wife Corinne (who was my girlfriend at the time) was about to leave to run some errands. I was sitting on a chair in our living room, when suddenly the entire universe was dissolved into Light. I felt weightless, shot through with joy beyond description. I loved everything. I was love. There was no individual *I* at all. Light poured from my eyes, from the pores of my skin. Corinne gasped, and wept, awestruck. And then the phone rang.

Some short time later, I went to meet this teacher, whose name is now GurujiMa. I sat with her in a room and she told me that she saw me in a prior life as a seeker in India, wandering with no possessions, living on pilgrimage, on the road, in caves, searching for truth. She drew me into myself, a self that extends beyond birth and death, into the endless reality that pervades all created things. The word that the Upanishads use for this reality is *brahman*, the vast.

After meeting with her, I could not speak. The inner reality that she introduced to me could not connect to my outer life, my personality. The gulf was too wide. During the nearly two decades since this meeting, my primary work has been bridging this divide. I have now had many experiences of this inner reality upon which my outer reality rests. I have walked back and forth across the bridge between inner and outer, sometimes immersed in the bliss of eternal joy, sometimes cut off and shrouded in the mist of isolation, unable to feel the inner reality at all. When I look back, I see that the gulf has narrowed, and these two worlds have begun to integrate. The chasm remains, but my experience of self is now native to both, and every breath joins them more.

> "The Upanishads are epic hymns of self-knowledge and world-knowledge and God-knowledge."
>
> The Upanishads by Sri Aurobindo

The *Upanishads* are profound crystallizations of immortal wisdom. They convey not ideas or concepts primarily, but experiences, and they do so in the form of revelatory poetry. The wisdom of the Upanishads can be found in philosophical threads throughout history, including the teachings of Buddha, Pythagoras, Plato, Gnosticism, Sufism, Metaphysics, the Transcendentalists, Theosophy, the New Age Movement, and the amalgam of ideas and beliefs that pervade the modern yoga community. The *Upanishads* transmit the core of spiritual mysticism, and so relate to the mystical streams of all spiritual traditions, and because they are non-religious and universalist in nature, their simple truths resonate across religious boundaries and divisions.

> *"[The Upanishads are] an expression of a mind in **which philosophy and religion and poetry** are made one, because **this religion** does not end with a cult nor is limited to a religio-ethical aspiration, but rises to an infinite discovery of God, of Self, of our highest and whole reality of spirit and being and speaks out of an ecstasy of luminous knowledge and an ecstasy of moved and fulfilled experience, **this philosophy** is not an abstract intellectual speculation about Truth or a structure of the logical intelligence, but Truth seen, felt, lived, held by the*

> *inmost mind and soul in the joy of utterance of an assured discovery and possession, and* **this poetry** *is the work of an aesthetic mind lifted up beyond its ordinary field to express the wonder and beauty of the rarest spiritual self-vision and the profoundest illumined truth of self and God and universe."*
>
> The Upanishads by Sri Aurobindo

In order to touch and be touched by these pearls of wisdom, we need to seek and find that within ourselves which resonates with them. The mind can take the words and concepts and interrogate and dissect them, looking for lines of logic, but then we will have missed the power and the beauty. We need to discover a faculty and an experience that is deeper and wiser than the mental, that can directly touch the rays of light that pour from the *Upanishads*.

> "It is because these seers saw Truth rather than merely thought it, clothed it indeed with a strong body of intuitive idea and disclosing image, but a body of ideal transparency through which we look into the illimitable, because they fathomed things in the light of self-existence and saw them with the eye of the Infinite, that their words remain always alive and immortal, of an inexhaustible significance, and inevitable authenticity, a satisfying finality that is at the same time an infinite commencement of truth, to which all our lines of investigation when they go through to their end arrive again and to which humanity constantly returns in its minds and its ages of greatest vision."
>
> The Upanishads by Sri Aurobindo

Context

The Vedas are each made up of four main parts. The *Samhitas* are the primary hymns of praise and communion that form the foundation of the *Vedas*. When someone refers to the *Rig Veda*, they are most likely referring to the *Rig Veda Samhita*. The next three parts are not clearly delineated – there is not absolute distinction between them, and often parts of them overlap and contain each other. The *Brahmanas* are commentaries on the hymns, mostly focused on the proper performance of rituals developed by an elite class of priests that emerged in the centuries after the original Vedic revelation. The Brahmanas are considered *karma-kanda*, or texts related to rituals. The *Aranyakas*, also developed by the new priestly caste, focus mainly on philosophical commentaries on the Vedic rituals, and along with the *Upanishads* are considered *jñāna-kanda*, or texts related to knowledge. The *Upanishads*, many of which are found as chapters within *Brahmanas* and *Aranyakas*, are condensed revelations of spiritual experience.

Upanishads are found throughout the four *Vedas* – the *Rigveda*, *Yajurveda*, *Sāmaveda*, and *Atharvaveda*. They build upon the Vedic symbolism discussed in previous chapters, and many of them include references to the *devas* and *asuras* – beings and forces of light and darkness around which the *Vedas* turn. But the crux of the *Upanishads* is the message that the universal cosmic Oneness that continually creates the universe, often called *brahman*, and the individual soul, often called ātman, are one. The ātman is not born with the human body, nor does it die, but moves through birth after birth in a flow of learning and deepening until its final liberation, or *moksha*. Throughout its journey, it experiences itself as separate from *brahman*, but this experience is caused by delusion and not actually true. This is the core of the philosophical tradition known as *Vedanta*, or the culmination of the *Vedas*.

There are hundreds of Upanishads, but the commonly accepted Muktika, or canon of liberation, includes 108. The list of Muktika Upanishads can be found here. Of the Muktika, 13 Upanishads are considered Mukhya, or principal. The list of Mukhya Upanishads can be found here.

Advaita Vedanta and Renunciation

In the centuries after the original *Upanishads* were written, many commentators used them as the basis for their philosophical doctrines. Among these, the most famous is Ādi Shankara, who lived during the 8th century in India. Shankara's doctrine became the school or lineage of *Advaita* (non-dual) *Vedanta*. His essential teaching was that *brahman* is the only reality, and totally identical with ātman. He argued that the physical world, in fact anything that is subject to change, is fundamentally illusory and unreal, or *māyā*. Essentially, there is only one actual reality and it is eternal, and anything that changes is false. The practical application of Shankara's teaching is renunciation, and throughout the years, countless ascetic monks, called *sannyasins* or *sādhus*, have left home, family, and all trappings of a personal life to seek liberation from the illusory world through meditation and austerities. Thousands of *sadhus* throughout India today belong to Shankara's order of ascetic monks and can be seen walking the streets of any town with a significant pilgrimage site.

Other commentators taught variations on Shankara's theme, and his commentaries have been argued over for centuries. Sri Aurobindo agrees with Shankara's assertion that ātman and *brahman* are one. He says, "The *brahman* alone is, and because of It all are, for all are the *brahman*." But he refutes the idea that everything that changes is unreal. Sri Aurobindo asserts that this evolutionary world in which we live, where life and mentality and consciousness itself are evolving and progressing, must have been intentional, for all that exists does so with the consent of the Divine One. This long and arduous adventure from ignorance and separation toward knowledge and union, from the dark night of isolation to the joyful re-union and rediscovery of the Divine Self in all, must be part of a plan that is wider than the human intelligence can perceive.

This teaching gives purpose to each of our lives, to our unique paths and to our originality. While an individual's life path may take one out of society and into silent contemplation for a limited or extensive time period, Sri Aurobindo does not believe that this path is the only real and true path for humanity. Our lives are not purposeless burdens that should be dropped so we can find liberation in the silence of the forest or a cave. That said, the internalization of the sannyasin archetype is a valuable aspect of any spiritual path. Instead of rejecting our outer lives, we can ask ourselves – what are we willing to let go of in order to seek liberation? Can we let go of attachment to our thoughts, our firmly held beliefs? Can we release entitlement to our emotions, reactions, and selfish desires? Can we let go of mental models that define reality in a limiting way, boxing it in to make it palatable? Can we let go of our judgments and attachment to seeing ourselves through the eyes of others? Can we let go of the shore and merge with the constant flow of creation that moves through us all the time?

Inner Reality: Trusting the Unseen

As we go within and explore our inner dimension, we begin to see that thought is not the final frontier. In fact, thoughts can be like clouds in the sky, blocking the sun's radiance. When we pay excessive attention to our thoughts, and allow them to solidify into rigid beliefs, we can develop a thick and unyielding personality that rejects vulnerability. And when we define ourselves based on others' judgments, this dense layer is reinforced and strengthened.

In order to see what's really there we need to soften, become vulnerable, and release the thoughts and beliefs that make up this coating. When we learn to yield our weight to the earth as we move around in our bodies, instead of propping ourselves up using our muscular strength, we gain resilience, relaxed stamina, and comfort. In the same way, when we learn to yield to the Divine One that encompasses and infuses us, letting our sense of self arise from this field of love rather than our habits and conditioning, we gain inner stability, integrity, and grace.

Each life is woven together into a vast fabric where every thought, prayer, word and action impacts the whole, and thus holds deep meaning. We are entirely integrated into the cosmos, so every movement of heart, mind or body that we make changes everything, including the movement to know ourselves. When we value our inner life, we encourage others to do the same, and support a collective movement toward greater authenticity. This takes commitment in a world that draws us out, encourages us to determine our self-worth based on the judgments of others, and see ourselves from the outside.

But we are meant to live from the inside out, not from the outside in. We are meant to live in the spontaneous and constant flow of truth that pours from the eternal and unchanging One into this world of change. As the truth that is love floods the world of form, all that resists truth is swept away by its irresistible current. This is the vast sweep of evolution, from the big bang to this moment and beyond into the miracle of tomorrow. It's where we are all headed together.

As a yoga teacher, students will come to you looking for both physical practice and practical philosophy, how to live comfortably in a body, and how to find purpose in their lives. In both areas you can only transmit to them what you have realized yourself. You can say all kinds of things, but they will be just words and ideas unless they are alive within you. Touching your inner landscape and valuing your inner experiences will enhance not only your own life but the lives of your students and everyone around you.

And progressing along our own inner journey of self-discovery, we join the Upanishadic sages who dove within in pursuit of the ultimate Truth, the ultimate Reality. The *Upanishads* are experienced realities, not abstract ideas. Our modern sensibilities struggle with the idea of a subjective truth that is realized within one's own inner world and is not easily objectively verifiable.

The scientific method is an amazing and profoundly valuable asset, as it encourages us to test our hypotheses rather than just believe whatever our thoughts or emotions serve up as truth. But it has become so synonymous with materialism that we think of something as verifiable only if it can be proven in the outer, physical world. The seers of the *Upanishads* surely used the scientific method – they tested and re-tested and shared and compared their experiences, but they did not depend on material reality as the sole definer of truth and reality.

We can do the same. Within us is a world that is complex and multidimensional, populated and penetrated by beings (devas and asuras and everything in between) and forces that seek to support our self-realization or lead us astray. Not everything we find can be trusted. We need to be rigorous in our self-seeking, but not with materialism as the proof. Love is the proof, the touchstone, the guiding light that illuminates our inner darkness. Not a superficial and selfish emotion that often passes for love in our modern world – but love that is wholeness, self-giving and self-nurturing, love that is unity and truth. This is the love that is yoga.

"Not a mere thinking and considering by the intelligence, the pursuit and grasping of a mental form of truth by the intellectual mind, but a seeing of it with the soul and a total living in it with the power of the inner being, a spiritual seizing by a kind of identification with the object of knowledge is jñāna. And because it is only by an integral knowing of the self that this kind of direct knowledge can be made complete, it was the self that the Vedantic sages sought to know, to live in and to be one with it by identity. And through this endeavor they came to easily see that this self again is the same as God and Brahman, a transcendent Being or Existence, and they beheld, felt, lived in the inmost truth of all things in the universe and the inmost truth of man's inner and outer existence by the light of this one and unifying vision."

The Upanishads by Sri Aurobindo

Purification

The *Pavamāna Abhyāroha* is a beautiful prayer that appears in the *Brihadaranyaka Upanishad* (1.3.28):

om asato mā sad gamaya,
tamaso mā jyotir gamaya,
mṛtyor mā amṛtaṃ gamaya
om śāntiḥ śāntiḥ śāntiḥ

Pavamāna is a word that appears throughout the *Rig Veda* in the context of purification. And *abhyāroha* has a sense of an ascending prayer of devotion. This prayer of purification is a calling out to be led (*gamaya*) from falsehood (*asat*) to truth (*sat*), from darkness (*tamas*) to light (*jyoti*), from death (*mrityu*) to immortality (*amrita*).

Purification is often misunderstood or misrepresented in modern western yoga. Part of this is because yoga today is frequently used to bolster the ego's false power. It's lumped in with fad diets and cosmetic surgery as a way to make us better, more lovable, worthier. We see what the ego does with the idea of purity and perfection, twisting it to strengthen the walls of its fortress. But true purification, like yoga, is not a means of strengthening the separated, isolated, lonely self. It's not a tool for self-improvement, but a process of profound self-love.

Looking back at yoga's history, we see traditions of self-mortification and self-denial that flowed from Shankara's doctrine of *māyā-vāda*. *Māyā-vāda* holds that all form is illusion, and that we should endeavor to escape the illusion by rejecting our bodies, our material lives, and our family/social ties to identify totally with the pure immortal oneness. Yogis in the *māyā-vāda* tradition leave society and practice self-deprivation and self-mortification (literally killing the self) as an approach to purification.

But the Divine One created this form and is this form. From the *Isha Upansihad*, "All this that moves within the moving universe is for the Lord's habitation." And the *Taittirriya Upanishad*, "Itself created itself; none other created it. And so it is called beautiful. And this that is beautifully made, it is no other than the Delight behind existence." If we reject the form of our bodies or the form of our lives as essentially illusory, then we reject that One Who is that form.

At the same time, we do find that we are immersed in falsehood. We are surrounded by confusion about what's real, what's true, what's good and wholesome. We live in an evolutionary universe where the Divine One is emerging from the depths of ignorance and separation toward the expanse of truth and unity. We are this evolution; our collective awakening is the re-union of the One Divine Beloved with itself in the form of many Divine Beloveds.

Spiritual purification is not self-destructive. It is loving and nurturing. If you find a child covered in blankets, suffocating beneath the weight, the most loving act is to begin taking off the layers that keep the child trapped. So it is with your essential self, or ātman. The ātman is the deepest and truest you, the one that is covered in blankets and aching to breathe and be free. And purification is the process of peeling away the layers of falsehood that obscure your natural radiance.

This requires discernment, but we need not face it alone. Prayer acknowledges that purification is a partnership between ātman and *Brahman*, between the individual and God. Without this partnership, we are left with the ego in charge. To paraphrase Ramana Mahārshi, when the thief is made the policeman, there will be plenty of investigation, but no arrests. Even as we experience ourselves as a limited individual self, enclosed within the walls of our own mind, we can call upon and receive support from the vast intelligent Love that holds all within its infinite heart.

Purification can happen on the level of the mind, the life, and the body. Purifying your mind does not require rejecting your mind; it requires discerning and releasing those thoughts, beliefs and ideas that are limiting, anti-love, and anti-life, including those that we cling to within ourselves and those that we take in through movies, books, "news" outlets, etc. Purifying your life does not require leaving behind your work, your family, your friends, and your home; it requires releasing those aspects of work, those relationships, and those attachments that are limiting, anti-love, and anti-life. Purifying your body not require rejecting it, denying its basic needs for food, water, movement, and breath; it requires releasing addiction and attachment to foods and drinks that harm the body and create confusion in the mind and emotions, and spending time listening to your body and its innate desire to move and breathe and laugh and cry.

The body in particular is a field of great promise and great challenge. In modern western culture it is common to live in a dis-embodied way, to live in our minds. Bringing awareness into the body is itself inherently an act of purification, especially when accompanied by prayer. The light of your awareness, joined with Divine Light, begins to penetrate the layers of obscurity held in the body, layers that are not just your own, but are part of the primal obscurity of matter. Entering the body, touching these layers can be uncomfortable. But staying with it, keeping the light of awareness in the body, exploring the layers of physicality and their innate wisdom and beauty, inherently clarifies and purifies the body and illuminates ways of loving and tending to its needs. Unwholesome desires become more obvious, and we can begin to let them go. Unloving behaviors stand out.

We can bring the light of our awareness into our bodies while we move. We can savor the experience of tending to the body, feeling the flow of life force seeping and rushing, pulsing and swirling to nourish and enliven our tissues, organs, glands and bones. Every aspect of the human body is holy, and it seeks to express its vibrancy. The body longs to radiate and join with the ātman in a pure expression of divinity. We can nurture this longing and draw the body and ātman into proximity, into relationship, and into yoga (union).

The reunion of the Divine One and the Divine Many takes place not in some theoretical cosmic realm. It takes place here, in your body, in your life, in your mind. And the best way of discerning whether you are heading in the right direction on the path of purification is love. Your heart has an innate ability to sense love. We need to release selfishness, fear and greed in order to activate and empower this sense, but it is a natural part of our embodiment. If you are unclear whether a certain belief or behavior is serving your growth toward wholeness, look for love. Don't look for ideas about love, look for the presence of love itself as a felt experience in your heart and it will lead you always toward truth and the purity of your own being.

"Beloved, lead us from falsehood to truth, from darkness to light, and from death to immortality." The *Pavamāna* prayer is not a rejection of life, but the innate and natural cry of the separated self to be joined with All. This longing for union fuels evolution. It transforms and progressively purifies your mind, your life, and your body. The body will become a true and pure home for the soul, not by destroying it or repressing its natural desires, but by releasing the desires that serve separation and not wholeness, enmity and not love. This process is collective and inevitable; it is the sweep of evolution. We can join in the flow, or we can be carried forward while we struggle and cling to the past. The path of purification frees us to let go of all that would hold us back and become the flow toward yoga, toward the embodiment of universal love.'

Seed Crystals of Truth

The reality touched by the ancient rishis blazes through their words with a crystallized intensity. Some passages are more difficult to access because of their symbolism, but some are quite direct and stark in their articulation. Here are just a few examples:

"You cannot see the seer of seeing; you cannot hear the hearer of hearing; you cannot think of the thinker of thinking; you cannot know the knower of knowing. This is your self that is within all; everything else but this is perishable."
– *Briha daranyaka Upanishad* 3.4.2

"Into a blind darkness they enter who follow after the Ignorance, they as if into greater darkness who devote themselves to Knowledge alone." – *Īsha Upanishad* 1.9

"That which thinks not by the mind, that by which the mind is thought, know That to be the Brahman and not this which men follow after here." – *Kena Upanishad* 1.5

"As the spider puts out and gathers in, as herbs spring up upon the earth, as hair of head and body grow from a living human, so here all is born from the Immutable." – *Katha Upanishad* 1.1.7

"I am one and unique in all respects. I am full, whole, and complete. I am pure, uncorrupt, and pristine. I am an image of deliverance and emancipation. I am free of all encumbrances and dark veils or coverings...I am without a birth. I am the supreme Truth personified. I am the essence of that truth and absolute reality." – *Ātmaprabadha Upanishad* 2.6

"This is the Self within my heart: smaller than a grain of rice...or a mustard seed, or a grain of millet, or the kernel of a grain of millet. This is the Self within my heart: more vast than the earth, more vast than the atmosphere, more vast than the heavens, more vast than all the worlds...This is the Self within my heart." – *Chandogya Upanishad* 3.14.3

In all their beauty and subtlety, perhaps the most valuable lesson we can take from the *Upanishads* is to value our inner experience. You are unique. You are original. And you are indivisible from the One Love that embraces all. To bring your uniqueness into the world requires understanding your inner landscape and all the helpers and obstacles that inhabit and travel within it. The rich and ancient yoga tradition speaks to us in a million verses on this same theme – go within, know yourself, and shine like the sun.

Chapter - 4

The Rāmāyana – Bhakti, Dhārma, and Karma

> *"Having polished the mirror of my heart with the dust from my guru's feet, I'll describe the spotless glory of Raghuvara (Ram), who bestows the four fruits of life."*
>
> from Sri Hanumān Chalīsa by Tulasidasa

It's our first night in the Kumaon Hills, the foothills of the majestic Himalayas, and I've been up the whole night with fever and diarrhea. I'm still kind of nauseous and feeling burned out, shaky. But I decide to make the trip to Kainchi, to Neem Karoli Baba's Ashram anyway. I feel drawn there despite my fatigue and dizziness. I hop into the back of the Land Rover, but after a few minutes on the bumpy roads that snake along the edges of deep ravines, switching back and forth as they ascend to passes and descend to valleys, I realize that I need to sit in the front. I suck on a ginger lozenge.

After a little over half an hour, we arrive, and I stand on the bridge that spans the rushing stream between Kainchi Ashram and the road. I look at the water pouring down toward me, and my heart reaches out to the Guru Maharaji Neem Karoli, who founded this ashram and passed from his body in 1973. "Why am I sick? What is this illness for?" I ask. "Fear. You are releasing fear," is the answer. It makes sense. The physical sensation of nausea and shakiness is similar to fear, anxiety, and it leads to worried thoughts about whether I'll get better, how I'll manage during this trip, what kind of terrible disease might be lurking within me, ready to gobble me up.

I cross the bridge and go sit in meditation facing the statue of Maharaji. I pray for clarity and guidance and protection. I offer my heart. And then I hear a commotion. I open my eyes, and a giant male monkey is sitting between me and Maharaji's statue. He looks into my eyes, bears his teeth, and reaches toward me. A nearby guard jumps to attention and fires a stone from his slingshot at the monkey, who screams and jumps, swinging himself up onto a ledge and out of sight. "That was a big one!" The guard smiles at me with a look of surprise. Yea. Wow. It has been said that Maharaji was an incarnation of Hanuman, the monkey who loved Ram above all else, and who was the embodiment of courageous faith and fierce devotion.

I close my eyes, and sink into the swirl of fear that surges through my body. I feel it, let it wash through me, and I offer it, release it, let it pour out into Maharaji's loving embrace. I sit for a long time with my fear, grateful for the loving force that draws it from me and offers comfort and reassurance. Maharaji's presence feels so personal, so close. The monkey's part in this play of life feels like a gift, a reminder that life is magical, mystical, that the rigid laws of science are just habits, waiting to be broken by a burst of divine drama.

Ādi-Kavya – The First Poem

Valmiki's 24,000 verse epic poem *Rāmāyana* is considered ādi-kavya, the first poem, in the yoga tradition. Modern scholarship assumes that it was written during the first few centuries BCE, but according to the story itself, it was written at the end of the *treta yuga*, around 800,000 years ago per Vedic cosmology.

The general sense of time in the yogic epics and legends conflicts significantly with our modern sense of history. But as the author Ramesh Menon says in *The Siva Purāna Retold*, "It is absurd that we pass any judgment whatever on a universe in which we are such infants: that we dare say 'This is so and this is not so in the cosmos'. Surely, our human history is an infinitesimal part of the history of the universe, not vice versa; and our ignorance is far more profound than our knowledge." Perhaps this kind of humility can help us keep an open mind as we explore stories taking place hundreds of thousands of years ago featuring fantastical creatures jumping across oceans, lifting mountains, and shooting arrows with the force of atomic bombs.

There are many versions of the essential *Rāmāyana* in various languages, and though a version of the original Sanskrit poem exists, it's unclear how much has been added or changed over the years. The first and seventh chapters in particular contain some narrative and stylistic contradictions with the rest of the text, as well as some controversial content, and they are assumed to have been added later.

The Story

The *Rāmāyana* chronicles the life of Ram, who was born the oldest of King Dasharatha's five sons, and heir to the throne. Rām is known by the narrator and some sages to be an *avatāra* (incarnation) of Lord Vishnu, the primordial Divine Being. He has come to the Earth to vanquish an evil *rākshasa* (demon) king named Rāvana who has conquered *prithvi* (Earth), *svarga* (Heaven), and *pātāla* (The Underworld). Rāvana has ten heads and fangs and feeds on human flesh. He practiced austerities for thousands of years and earned a boon from the Creator Brahmā, who granted that no *deva* (celestial being) could kill him. When Rāvana conquered *svarga*, he kicked out all the *devas* that hadn't been slain in battle, and they were forced to wander the three worlds, hiding and trembling in fear. They came to Lord Vishnu, praying for his mercy, and he agreed to incarnate as a man to slay Rāvana. This man was Rām.

> *"Perceiving that the devas and the Earth were terror-stricken and hearing their loving entreaties, a solemn voice came from heaven which dispelled their doubt and anxiety: 'Fear not, O sages, adepts and devas! For your sake, I will assume the form of a man with every element of my divinity...I shall relieve the Earth of all its burden; be fearless O devas.'"*
>
> from Sri Ramacharitamanasa by Tulasidasa

Rām was a divine incarnation of beauty, righteousness, and truth. But being immersed in a limited human form, he suffered as humans do, experiencing grief, despair, and fear. When Rām's coronation is imminent, his step-mother Kaikeyi calls upon King Dasharatha to fulfill an old promise that he had made to grant her anything in the world she might request. He agrees, and she asks that her son Bhārat be made king, and that Rām be banished to the forest for fourteen years. When Kaikeyi speaks the words, Dasharatha collapses to the floor. He knows that he cannot take back his word, but he is so devastated by her request that after Rām leaves for the forest, he dies of a broken heart. Even Bhārat himself tries to convince Rām to just take the throne anyway, but his commitment to truth is total. He cannot dishonor his father's word.

Rām is joined in his exile by his wife Sīta and his brother Lakshman, both of whom follow him into the forest despite his protests. One day, Sīta spots a beautiful deer and asks Rām to catch it for her. The deer is actually one of Rāvana's spies in disguise. When Rām wanders far into the forest, and then Lakshman goes to look for him, Rāvana captures Sīta, flies her on his spaceship to Lanka, and imprisons her in the Ashoka Grove near his palace.

When Rām returns to find Sītā missing, he collapses in despair. Lakshman comforts him, and together they begin the search for Sītā. They receive help from Jatāyū, a great ancient vulture who saw Rāvana escaping with Sītā and fought with him. Rām and Lakshman come upon Jatāyū laying nearly dead on the ground, and he tells them that Rāvana has taken Sītā south. They set out, and their journey leads them through the forests to a kingdom of *vānaras* (literally forest people, but with vast strength and monkey-like hair and tails). Among the *vānaras* Rām and Lakshman meet Hanumān, who is destined to play a big role in reuniting Rām and Sītā.

From the moment he meets Ram, Hanumān recognizes him as the Divine Beloved, and surrenders himself entirely in service to him. The Rāmāyana's fifth chapter is called the *Sundara Khanda* (literally *beautiful episode*), and illustrates Hanumān's leap across the ocean to Lanka in search of Sītā. He finds her and gives her Ram's ring, bringing a light of hope to her dark situation. Hanumān then allows himself to be captured by Rāvana so he can investigate, and when Rāvana's guards light Hanumān's tail on fire to torture him, he breaks free and jumps from roof to roof, igniting the city and burning much of it to the ground.

There is a moment at the beginning of the *Sundara Khanda* when Hanumān is sitting atop a mountain by the seashore, looking out over the vast ocean. He has been chosen by his friends to make the leap to Lanka in search of Sītā, but he doubts himself. When he was young his super powers got him into trouble, so Indra, Lord of Heaven, made him forget his true nature to keep him contained. Now he faces his doubts, and then dives within to find the source and depth of his strength. He longs to be of service, and he has been shown the path of his *dharma*, but he feels his own limitations, and he is afraid.

After Hanumān returns and confirms that Sītā is in fact imprisoned on Lanka, Rāma invokes Varuna, god of the sea, and asks him to allow them passage to Lanka. Varuna assures Rām that if the *vānara* Nala builds a bridge, it will not sink. The bridge is built, and the army of *vānaras* crosses over with Rām and Lakshman leading. The epic battle between the *vānaras* and the *rākshasas* is described in intense detail, and in the end Rāvana lays dead with Rām's arrow through his heart.

Rāvana

Rāvana kidnapped Sītā because he heard that she was the most beautiful woman in the world. Having conquered the three worlds and established his rule, Rāvana was still hungry. From the moment that he decided to kidnap Sītā until the time of his death, he was warned countless times by his own advisors, his spies, his own brother, and of course by Hanumān, that Rām would destroy him. He seemed even to know it in his own heart by the end, but he was unable to let Sītā go. He mistook lust for love, and he believed that he could control Sītā and compel her to be what she was not, to forsake her *dharma* for a false life as his queen.

Rāvana was a great king, an incomparable scholar, a yogi, a healer, and a brilliant musician. But he held within him an essential darkness that has inhabited man and his relationship to woman for thousands of years. This darkness deludes man into believing that love is control, that strength is domination, and that lust is love. Immense suffering has flowed from this one distortion, which is at the very beginning stages of unraveling today. We have a long way to go, but the world is beginning to wake up and see that Rāvana's greed masks a profound loneliness that cannot be met by Sītā. Sītā's fidelity and refusal to give him what he wants was a profound gift to Rāvana, as it invited him to face the roots of his pain. The gaping ache can only be filled by Rāvana discovering his true nature as a child of God. It is said that because he was killed by Rām, after his death Rāvana attained the state of highest liberation and was eternally freed from suffering. Sīta's steadfastness and Rām's grace liberated him.

Bhakti

Hanumān is revered in the yogic tradition as an embodiment of courage and faith. The Hanumān Chalīsa is a widely popular prayer written by the saint Tulsidas, himself considered an incarnation of the original Rāmāyana's author (Valmiki). It was written in Awadi, a variant of Hindi, and it consists of forty verses in praise of Hanumān. There is a popular addendum to the Rāmāyana in which Rām gives Hanumān a gold ring as they fly back home after the battle with Rāvana. Hanumān immediately throws the ring into the ocean, saying that he won't accept anything that doesn't have Ram's name on it. Someone points out that Hanumān's body doesn't have Ram's name on it, and he rips open his chest, revealing Rām and Sīta radiating from within his heart. This link offers a version of the story told by my friend Peter Malakoff.

This kind of devotion to an embodied being is often met with skepticism in the modern west, but Hanumān is revered as the ultimate role model throughout India. In giving himself entirely to Rām's service, he embodies the path of *Bhakti* Yoga, the yoga of devotion. *Bhakti* is a path to union with the Divine that centers on the heart, and on uplifting and purifying all human emotionality through the fire of divine love. Love for God is something natural and innate in all humans, even though it's often hidden from our daily experience. *Bhakti* practices focus on uncovering this love by chanting the names of God's many incarnations and emanations, telling stories about God's graceful interventions in human affairs, and meditating on God's qualities.

The natural relationship of a part to its whole is devotion, reverence, and love. A fruit naturally worships the tree from which it grows, a tree loves the forest that nourishes it, and a forest resonates with gratitude and bhakti for the Earth. God is our source, and the whole that comprises all our innate honoring of the Divine Beloved is not something that we fabricate or contrive. We discover it by removing the layers of false beliefs, fear, and coping mechanisms that we have developed to deal with the experience of separation.

When we incarnated as humans on Earth, we left the experience of infinite oneness with the source of our being; we left the experience of being upheld and supported and surrounded by love. That reality is still within us, but it's buried, and we have turned to behaviors that seem to approximate that experience of comfort and belonging, but in reality don't provide true satisfaction. These behaviors become addictions to relationships, to control, to distraction, to getting high on adrenaline, drugs and drama. Releasing these coping mechanisms and seeking for something invisible requires courage, perseverance, and faith.

Hanumān's father was Vāyu, the god of the wind. He is called Pāvanaputra, or son of the wind, and his father Vāyu helps him make the impossible leap across the ocean to Lanka. The great 20th century yogi Neem Karoli Baba, who is said to have been an incarnation of Hanumān, called him "the breath of Rām." God's breath is always with us, flowing through us, flowing through life. Just as Hanumān leapt across the ocean to remind Sītā that her beloved Rām was seeking her, God's breath pours from the heart of the cosmos into our bodies, reminding us that our Beloved is near.

Sītā

Sītā was also a divine incarnation, an embodiment of the Divine Mother. Her name means "furrow," and she is a daughter of the

Earth, found in a field by her father King Janaka. The Mother of the Universe is born as Daughter of the Earth to heal the Earth through the offering of her pain. While on the surface of the story, it was Rām that stormed Rāvana's island with his army and ultimately shot an arrow through his heart, he was acting on Sītā's behalf. Sītā endured Rāvana's lustful advances, his seductions, and his aggression because she had faith in Rām. She understood that she couldn't physically overcome the demon herself, but when she had the opportunity to escape she did not take it, knowing that Rāvana's destiny was to fall by Rām's hand.

How many times in a day do we face the choice to push forward with our own will or wait in faith for God to act? Sītā was confronted by an enormous ten-headed monster with fangs who threatened to eat her if she didn't become his wife. Our circumstances are usually much milder, and yet the inclination to fight or flee is strong. Waiting in faith, even if we see clearly that it's the right course, can feel like trying to hold back a freight train. And yet God is always with us, holding every situation, preparing to intervene when the time is right. We don't allow space for divine action, and we don't appreciate it when it doesn't match our expectations or fulfill our myopic desires.

Dhārma

Rām embodies *dhārma*, which is a term that's difficult to translate into English, but carries the sense of right action/living, alignment with truth and righteousness, and sacred purpose. It is often narrowly translated as *duty* or *law*, but this understanding of the word leaves out the spiritual dimension that supersedes human concepts of morality. Divine law defies formulation or rigidity. It must be received rather than conceptualized, and we need a way to suspend our thoughts and beliefs and judgments and enter into relationship with the flow of God's breath.

We need a practice of inner alignment in which we sit, align all layers of our self, and open to sensing spiritual *dhārma* as it unfolds now. As soon as we start strategizing or judging, worrying or regretting, grasping or clenching, we've stepped out of the stream. A practice of alignment allows the emergent *dhārma* of the present moment to pour through us and inspire action that serves the highest purposes of our life. In asana practice we seek alignment so that prana can flow freely through our bodies, and a practice of inner alignment does the same thing. It takes us out of the patterns of prop and collapse that we've developed in life and into a state where truth and love can flow through us and into the world.

The truth is infinite and eternal, and our human minds are finite and limited. We tend to receive inspiration from the Divine and then immediately translate it to make it comprehensible by our limited minds. We are addicted to knowing, and will latch onto any idea that gives us the comfort of feeling that we know what will come tomorrow. The prayer "Thy will be done" is an alternative to this. Instead of trying to anticipate and control the future, or figure out what path to take, how to move forward in life, we can offer ourselves to the Divine and ask that Divine Will shape our life. The prayer itself purifies our consciousness, releasing all that would grasp for control. It invites the infinite wisdom that has given birth to countless galaxies to enter the infinitesimal circumstances of daily life and carry us forward.

There are several times during the Rāmāyana where Rām could have easily justified a decision based on human reasoning that would have made his life easier. In fact, he was encouraged to do so by just about everyone close to him. It's actually interesting just how much nuance and attention Valmiki gives to Rām's facing reasonable and rational arguments over and over again that conflict with his *dhārma*. But his answer is always the same.

To his brother Lakshman he says, "I must go to the forest, my fate lies there," and "The way of the soul is longer than fourteen years in a forest." To his mother, Kausalya he says, "The path I mean to tread leads straight to heaven, and any other to ruin." When his father asks him to stay for just one more night before departing, he replies "If I stay tonight, tomorrow you will ask me to stay another day. But I have already gone, for my spirit is on its way." When his brother Bhārata journeys for days in the forest to find him and ask him to return and take the crown, he says, "There was never any error in what has happened Bhārata. There are deeper forces at work in our lives than we know. There are greater tasks to be accomplished than we yet understand," and "I grant that common sense may cry out otherwise, but fate is beyond mere common sense." (These quotes are from The Rāmāyana, A Modern Retelling of the Great Indian Epic by Ramesh Menon.)

Rām remained committed to moving from his inner sense of truth, his inner guidance. He had a sense that he was being led somewhere important by a path that concealed its destination, and he persevered on that path. His decision was not rooted in rationality, nor was it rooted in sub-rational emotions. Ram's sense of *dharma* was supra-rational, more encompassing than mental reasoning. It flowed through him from the One Divine Heart of the Universe.

All humans have a unique *svadharma* that corresponds to their unique nature, constitution, *karma* and inclinations. As an avatar, Ram's *svadharma* has universal implications, but it is still his own path, and it is imprinted in him. Such is his nature that he cannot deviate from his *dharma*, even though that involves great pain for him and those he loves. We each are faced with the same archetype. An unseen hand guides us along a path that leads into the unknown, and every day we face the choice to remain faithful to our inner guidance or capitulate to voices of fear and mistrust that appeal to our rationality and reason. The society we live in constantly inundates us with the message that there is no spiritual reality underlying what we see and touch, that our daily life has no deeper purpose, and that we must be in control or be destroyed. Our minds absorb these ideas and they solidify into beliefs, the walls of our own private fortress. Then we wonder why we feel so depressed and lonely.

Karma

The *Uttara Kanda*, the seventh and final chapter of the *Rāmāyana*, contains a kind of postscript that details the karmic entanglements that led to the story's main events. The sage Valmiki reveals a complex web of interconnections spanning many lifetimes that links Ram, Sītā, Hanumān, Rāvana, and many of the other characters. Even the devas are subject to the process of karmic unfoldment.

In this evolutionary world where everything is consistently progressing toward wholeness, and truth is constantly expanding and exposing layer after layer of falsehood, karma is the process that supports this evolution. Every action that takes us away from wholeness and truth plants a seed, and each seed inevitably grows and bears fruit. The fruit may be sweet or bitter, but it always serves to advance our yoga – carrying us toward reunion with our entire self.

Karmas may take effect within a lifetime, or carry over from lifetime to lifetime, leaving the human self bewildered as to the source of misfortune. We look for something we've done to deserve our fate, and decide that our suffering must be a product of a chaotic and purposeless universe. But how could this majestic, intricate, delicately woven universe exist for no purpose? How could humanity have evolved from stardust and bacteria by chance? Just because we can't see the connections that carry through from one incarnation to another does not mean they are not there. Every action bears fruit in time, and every soul is on a long-term journey of self-discovery that can only end in the arms of absolute wholeness.

What if we experienced every circumstance in our lives, even the most painful ones, as gifts of love whose purpose is to nurture our growth toward wholeness? Every gain, every loss, every ache, every fall, every victory, every defeat is an opportunity for reconciliation and redemption. When we constantly run from the pain in our hearts, seeking distraction or deflection, the power of karmic healing is limited. But if we can bear the pain and sit with it, patiently allow it to unfold like a flower and reveal its hidden gifts, when it passes it takes with it a knot that has held us captive in some way. Every entanglement that we release leaves us a bit more free.

This is one of the principle messages of the *Rāmāyana*: God is real, acting in the world, and working always to set us free. Our faith and patience, our capacity to listen with discernment for guidance and courage to act when it arrives, and our attunement to the sweet breath of love that surrounds us all support a process of growth that is encoded into the fabric of the universe. Every moment of our lives, every breath is imbued with purpose for ourselves and for the entire Earth of which we are part. As we awaken to this reality, God's capacity to work in our lives increases, and miracles fall like rain and blossom like spring flowers.

> *"I worship him whose body is dark and beautiful like a rain-bearing cloud teeming with abundant delights;...with a pair of large lotus eyes and a tuft of matted locks on his head; the most glorious Rama, the delighter of all, traveling in the company of Sīta and Lakshmana."*
>
> from Sri Rāmacharitamānasa by Tulasidāsa

Chapter - 5

Sankhya Kārikā – Enumerating Reality

During the summer of 2001, I spent four months living high in the Eastern Sierras in California, rock climbing, backpacking, and working at a fishing lodge. As fall set in and the weather turned colder I traveled to the coast and joined a yoga program at the Mount Madonna Center outside of Santa Cruz. It was founded by the students of Baba Hari Das, who still lived and taught there at the time I arrived. When the prominent western yogi Ram Das was living with his guru Neem Karoli Baba in Kainchi in the Himalayan Foothills, Baba Hari Das was assigned to be his yoga teacher. His photo appears in the iconic book *Be Here Now*, and he was the architect of the beautiful Hanumangarh Temple in Nainital. When I met him, he was an elderly yogi with a long white beard who hadn't spoken a word in 50 years.

Baba Hari Das used a chalkboard to communicate, and his silence was a yogic commitment, or *sankalpa*. He had been a yogi for most of his seventy-eight years, having left home at the age of eight to attend a yoga school, and then officially renouncing the world as a sannyasi at the age of nineteen. He would give teachings on pranayama and Sankhya philosophy, using his chalkboard and a volunteer who would read the scribblings to the class. Having lived in Auroville and been exposed to the teachings of Sri Aurobindo and the Mother the year before, this was my introduction to what might be called Classical Yoga, as well as my first experience of sitting with a person who had dedicated their entire life to the practice and teaching of yoga.

In addition to teaching, Baba Hari Das would work with the crews building walls, buildings, statues. Even though he had renounced the typical life of a householder, he had not renounced action. He worked, practicing karma yoga. He spoke of striving for the action to be selfless, an offering of service given to life itself, without entitlement to the fruits of the action. Don't worry, he would say, just do the work.

And when it was time for the annual celebration of Navaratri, he fully participated in building the giant effigy of the demon king Ravana, which was set up in a field behind the ashram. On the last night of Navaratri, when we celebrated Rama's victory over Ravana and the essential victory of light over darkness, we gathered in front of this giant Ravana and watched as a burning arrow was shot through the air and into his belly, igniting the figure in a blaze of fire. We chanted and danced and jumped over the flames, and Baba was there through it all.

Baba Hari Das was a living example of yoga, and being with him simplified the complex teachings. He simply embodied his own perspective on what he had learned. The teachings themselves, especially when we get into the realm of *Sankhya* philosophy and the other five *darśanas*, is complex. These next two chapters are quite dense, and contain a great many concepts and a lot of Sanskrit words. I invite you to take them in and absorb what you can without feeling pressure to understand everything conceptually or memorize all the terms. Understanding grows organically with exposure over time, and I'm just offering a place to dip in and experience the flavor of these teachings. The teachings themselves were the framework for a lifetime of study, and what I'm hoping to provide is enough of an intro to honor the traditions themselves.

Six Darśanas

Within the lineage of Vedic spirituality, there are six recognized systems or schools of thought. They represent six branches of the river of yogic wisdom that has flowed since ancient times, from the distant past into the present. These were not competing schools, though sometimes their proponents have engaged in rhetorical argument. They were complimentary, and often shared and borrowed ideas, concepts, inquiries and perspectives from each other.

The metaphor of a river is especially appropriate: a river of wisdom flowing across the landscape of ancient India, branching off, reconverging, splintering, pouring over waterfalls, and carving out pools, ponds and lakes. A person's thirst for knowledge and understanding could be quenched by the water in any of these forms, as it was the same water. But its flavor might be different based on the unique soil and landscape through which it flowed.

These six systems are called the āstika *darśanas*. Āstika is generally translated as *orthodox*, but it literally means something more like *it exists*, the *it* being the *atman* or individual soul. So āstika systems recognize the existence of the individual soul. All six schools emerged after the Vedas themselves, and each accepts the Vedas as the ultimate spiritual authority. *Darśana* means *view of the truth*, and the *darśanas* are ways of understanding reality.

In addition to the six āstika *darśanas*, there were also *nāstika*, or unorthodox *darśanas* in ancient India, including Buddhism and Jainism. These systems did not accept the ultimate reality of the atman, nor did they recognize the authority of the Vedas, but their waters too have mixed and mingled with the six āstika *darśanas* to produce countless rivulets and pools of inquiry and wisdom.

This is why what we call 'yoga philosophy' can seem so daunting, confusing, and illusive. It's why different ideas seem to contradict each other. There is not just one stream of teaching that can be followed from origin to today, but thousands and millions of streams, passing through thousands and millions of individual teacher-student relationships. Some teachings emerged as major texts, some were lost to history. But always there was cross-pollination, interweaving of ideas and explorations and discoveries.

The six recognized āstika *darśanas* are *Sankhya, Yoga, Vaiśeshika, Nyāya, Mīmānsā,* and *Vedānta*. Each system has a distinct philosophical and cosmological perspective and approach, and has produced specific texts that align with its tenets. And while there are traditions and lineages associated with these six, most *gurus* historically would have been versed in several if not all of them. They would have merged and synthesized the collective wisdom with their own individual predilections and the influence of their environment and their culture, weaving teachings with the intention to help their students find liberation. And the same is true today: when people speak of 'yoga philosophy' today, they are weaving a tapestry, often using strands from both āstika and *nāstika darśanas*, woven together with the prevalent assumptions and needs of our current moment in time.

Six Pramānas

Each of the āstika *darśanas* has its own epistemology, or *pramāna*. A *pramāna* is basically an accepted way of distinguishing what is real from what is not. There are six *pramānas* in all, but each *darśana* accepts its own combination of them.

The six *pramānas* are:
Pratyaksha – direct perception
Anumāna – inference
Śabda – reliable testimony
Upamāna – comparison/analogy
Arthāpatti – hypothesis/conjecture
Anupalabdi – non-perception/negative proof

And the six *darśanas* with their corresponding *pramānas* are:
Sankhya – *pratyaksha, anumāna, and śabda*
Yoga – *pratyaksha, anumāna, and śabda*
Vaiśeshika – *pratyaksha and anumāna*
Nyāya – *pratyaksha, anumāna, śabda, and upamāna*
Mīmānsā - *pratyaksha, anumāna, śabda, upamāna, and athāpatti*
Vedānta - *pratyaksha, anumāna, śabda, upamāna, athāpatti, and anupalabdi*

For example, *Sankhya* and *Yoga* both say that you can know whether something is real or not by direct perception, inference, and reliable testimony.

Let's say you want to prove to your friend that it is raining. One way to do that would be to allow them to directly experience the rain: to see it, hear it, or feel it. This is *pratyaksha*. But let's say you want to prove that it's raining at the top of a mountain when you're at the bottom. You might show your friend a stream running down from the top of the mountain growing larger and faster. This is *anumāna*. What if you want to prove that it's raining in San Francisco? You might visit a reliable news website. This would be śabda. Śabda does hinge on the word *reliable*, which introduces some grey into the equation, but generally it is referring to scriptures that are considered to be of divine origin or awakened beings whose articulation of truth is one with the divine word.

Upamāna means comparison, or analogy. This pramāna says that you can know that something is real through its similarity to another thing that you know is real. So, if your friend had never seen snow before, but they had seen rain and ice, they could understand the concept of snow as a plausible reality based on its similarity to rain and ice.

Arthāpatti means hypothesis or conjecture. So perhaps you and your friend notice that earth and sky are dry before you go to sleep. Then when you wake up, you step outside and see wet earth, dripping leaves, and puddles. You can use arthāpatti to state that it rained during the night. You may notice that both upamāna and arthāpatti seem similar to anumāna. It's true, and the Sankhya, Yoga, and Nyāya darśanas all consider these two pramānas to be types of anumāna.

Anupalabdi means non-perception or negative proof. You take your friend by the hand, walk outside, and say "It's not raining." "How do you know?" your friend asks. "I don't see rain, I don't hear it, I don't feel it, and I don't smell or taste it, so I am sure there is an absence of rain." At any given time and place, rain either is present or absent. Anupalabdi provides a way of asserting the absence of a thing in a particular place at a particular time.

A traditional jñana yoga approach developed by Vedanta darśana involves investigating every aspect of inner and outer reality and asking "Is this real?" Am I my personality? Am I my liver? Am I my gut bacteria? Am I my memories? Am I my thoughts?" As we follow this inquiry deeper and deeper, we discard elements that we ordinarily assume to be real, static and lasting, until we arrive at nothing, a primordial emptiness. Anupalabdi supports this investigation, providing a way to prove that something does not exist.

Sankhya Darśana

Sankhya means enumeration, or inventory. This *darśana* is the oldest of the six, and it lays out a list of the fundamental elements of existence, or *tattwas*. The essential elements out of which all the rest arise are *purusha*, or spirit, and *prakriti*, matter. *Purusha* and *prakriti* are understood to be distinctly separate, neither one evolving from the other. The ultimate aim in the *Sankhya darśana* is to realize and merge with *purusha*, leaving behind the delusion of identification with *prakriti*, implying that *moksha*, or liberation from suffering, can be attained through *jñana*, or knowledge. When we know our true selves as pure spirit, we are free from the pain of identifying with the body and the environment that it relies upon.

The oldest known text of the *Sankhya darśana* is called the *Sankhya Kārikā*. The text itself refers to older *Sankhya* texts, so it is understood not to be the root text of the tradition, but a summary that was compiled probably during the first few centuries BCE. The *Sankhya Kārikā* is a collection of seventy-two metrical verses, and it begins by stating its purpose in the first *Kārikā*: "This is an inquiry into the prevention of suffering."

Yoga is primarily an intentional self-inquiry: Who am I? What is this which is not me, but which surrounds me? Where did I come from? Where am I going? Why do I suffer? How can I find peace? These are the fundamental questions of yoga, questions that are explored and expanded on through countless texts and commentaries by innumerable authors. They are explored through poetry, song, dance, painting, logic, story, and all possible means, dissected and reconstructed, probed and worshiped. The project of self-inquiry is the basic human project, one that we all share.

And this is the basis of the *Sankhya Kārikā*: an inquiry into the prevention of suffering, which, as the first verse goes on to state, is worthwhile because the usual methods of addressing suffering haven't given us lasting results. We need to take the inquiry deeper and understand where we come from and of what we are comprised. We will return to a deeper exploration of the *Sankhya Kārikā* after briefly touching on the other five darśanas.

Yoga Darśana

Yoga darśana has its roots in *Sankhya*, building upon its foundation and incorporating additional elements. While *Sankhya* describes the cosmos and its basic elements, *Yoga* points to the individual's relationship to the cosmos and the question of how to expand our own vision and understanding.

Yoga darśana leans heavily on its description of the cosmos as made up of 25 essential *tattwas*, and agrees that *moksha* is attainable through *jñana*. But *Yoga darśana* adds a moral code and set of specific techniques as a means of developing *jñana*. And *Yoga* also incorporates the honoring of the divine being called Īshvara, literally the Lord, and surrendering to Īshvara is included as one of the means of attaining *moksha*. *Yoga darśana* has actually been called "*Sankhya* with Īśvara", implying that it's essentially the same as *Sankhya* except for the inclusion of the Divine Lord as a cosmological component.

The primary early texts of *Yoga darśana* are the *Yoga Sūtra of Patañjali* and *Yoga Yajñavalkya*, but more recent texts like the *Hatha Yoga Pradipika*, the *Gheranda Samhita*, and the *Siva Samhita* are usually included in the *Yoga* lineage. We will discuss the *Yoga Sūtra* in depth in the next chapter.

Vaiśeshika Darśana

The *Vaiśeshika darśana* accepts only the first two *pramānas* as valid. But it skirts this edge a bit by including forms of testimony and analogy as variants of *anumāna*: not specific unique *pramānas* unto themselves, but types of inference.

Vaiśeshika is atomistic, and asserts that everything in the physical universe is made up of indestructible, indivisible, tiny atoms. Earth, water, fire and air are all material, and thus composed of atoms. Ether is material but infinite. And space, time, soul and mind are all infinite, eternal and immaterial. They are not composed of atoms but form the substrata of the material universe. According to *Vaiśeshika*, we can achieve the *jñana* (knowledge) that leads to *moksha* (liberation) when we thoroughly understand the world and how its constituent parts combine and interact.

Kanāda's *Vaiśeshika Sūtra* is the primary text of *Vaiśeshika darśana*, and additional texts include *Padārtha Dharmasangraha* and *Vyomavatī*, which offer both commentary on the original work and new and independent material.

Nyāya Darśana

Nyaya means something like right judgment, or correct rules. It was this *darśana* that developed India's fundamental system of logic. *Nyāya* aligns closely with *Vaiśeshika darśana*, and agrees that we find freedom from suffering through correctly understanding the universe. But it emphasizes that our general, superficial understanding of the world relies on assumptions and faulty logic.

To know something truly, we need to rigorously analyze our understanding, subjecting our rationality to *anuvyavasāya*, or metacognition. We have to think about our thoughts, reason through our reasons. The *Nyāya Sūtra* and *Nyāyavārttikatātparyaṭīkā* are two root texts of *Nyāya darśana*.

Mīmānsā Darśana

Mīmānsā darśana is an approach to understanding the Vedas, which it accepts as authorless and eternal. *Mīmānsā* means something like *consideration*, or *desire to think*. This *darśana* seeks to understand the nature of right action, or *dharma*. It differs from the other *darśanas* by asserting that without action, knowledge is useless. Happiness and the fulfillment of human destiny depend upon right action, and so we need to understand the nature of right action in order to free ourselves from suffering.

Mīmānsā darśana relies on the Vedas as the ultimate foundational eternal truth, and its basic approach is to dissect and inspect the Vedas, specifically focusing on everything that they have to say about *dharma*. It divides the passages of the Vedic texts into hymns, names, injunctions/commands, prohibitions and explanations, and uses these categories to extract the means of right living. Some commands and prohibitions are specifically related to Vedic rituals and which mantras to use in which combination at which times, and some are more about how to live and what kinds of behaviors are acceptable or unacceptable, killing cows or brahmins being examples of unacceptable behavior.

Overall, *Mīmānsā* can be said to be a collective summary of the rules and regulations for interpreting and understanding the Vedas and applying this understanding to life. And its goal is not liberation through contemplation, but salvation through fulfilling one's duty and purpose in life. As the *Sankhya Kārikā* begins with a definition of its aim to overcome suffering, the *Mīmānsāsūtra* begins with the statement "Now is the inquiry of *dharma*."

Vedānta Darśana

The sixth *darśana* is *Vedānta*. *Vedānta* is the most developed and best known (within India) of the six *darśanas*. It is sometimes called *Uttaramīmānsā*, which like *Vedānta* essentially has the connotation of the last, or ultimate understanding of the Vedas. *Vedānta* has several sub-*darśanas*, running the spectrum between *advaita* on one end and *dvaita* on the other. *Dvaita* means dual, and these sub-schools propose, similarly to *Sankhya*, a distinct split between spirit and matter. The schools of *Advaita Vedānta* are non-dual, and say that there is no distinction at all between *purusha* and *prakriti*, as matter is just a reflection of the eternal, primordial spirit. *Advaita Vedanta* is sometimes called Śārīrakamamīmānsā, or inquiry into the embodied spirit.

The primary text of *Vedanta* is the *Vedāntasūtra*, also called the *Brahmasūtra* because its primary focus is *brahman*, or the spiritual reality that permeates the universe and infuses all of existence. The *Vedāntasūtra* integrates the teachings of the *Upanishads*, which are themselves the second major text (or collection of texts) of *Vedānta*. An example of a theme that *Vedānta* draws from the *Upanishads* is the relationship between *brahman*, the fundamental reality that pervades and animates the cosmos, and *atman*, the individual soul. *Vedānta* concludes that *atman* and *brahman* are one and the same, one reality in two forms. This universal principle uniting the microcosm and the macrocosm, the individual and the cosmos, has been hugely influential throughout the history of yogic seeking, right up to the present day.

The third primary text of *Vedānta* is the *Bhagavad Gītā*, and Vedantic teachers and scholars assert the fundamental truth of these three texts (*Vedāntasūtra*, the *Upanishads*, and the *Bhagavad Gītā*) and seek to draw out their essential and relevant teachings and apply them to the particular milieus of their times. Together, the three texts are called the *prasthanātrayī*, or the three sources.

Sankhya Kārikā

Now that we've explored each of the six *darśanas* and their approach to understanding reality, let's go back to the earliest and most foundational of the six. *Sankhya darśana* provides a picture of the universe that all of the other *darśanas* build upon, and if we want to understand the roots of yoga and the framework that the lineages of yoga use, we need to understand this picture of the universe. *Patañjali's Yoga Sūtra*, for example, incorporates the twenty-five *tattwas* (fundamental elements of manifest reality) enumerated in the *Sankhya Kārikā*, and the eight limbs of yoga that we hear so much about in the modern yoga world rest on the foundation of *Sankhya* cosmology.

The *Sankhya Kārikā* begins by stating that its purpose is to explore the prevention of the "three-fold suffering." It characterizes suffering as being:

Ādhyātmika – arising from the body/mind system

Ādhibautika – arising from interactions with our environment, other people, animals, etc.

Ādhidaivika – arising from supernatural causes, including astrological and spiritual

And then it essentially says, "If you think that this effort to prevent pain is unnecessary because we already have the Vedas and they explain everything, then just look around and see if our understanding of the Vedas have permanently erased suffering. It might go away for a little while, but then it comes back. And the reason for that is that our relationship to the Vedas has become all tangled up with impurity, decay, and excess. What we need to do is to try to understand these three: the manifest reality, the unmanifest reality, and the knower."

And then the enumeration begins. *Kārikā* 3 lays out the *tattwas* initially, saying that, to begin with, we've got the primal nature, the source or root of all creation, *prakriti*, which does not evolve from anything. Then we've got seven *tattwas* that both evolve from somewhere and give rise to other *tattwas*. Sixteen more *tattwas* evolve from other *tattwas*, but don't themselves give rise to anything. And finally there is *purusha*, the pure spirit, which neither evolves from anything nor gives rise to anything. It is free and not at all involved in the whole chain of evolution that begins with *prakriti*.

After going through the *pramānas* that *Sankhya* accepts, basically laying out the rules of play, the text begins by articulating the fundamental differences between *purusha* and *prakriti*.

Prakriti and Purusha

Everything in the visible universe evolves from *prakriti*. It is the uncaused cause that must exist, *Sankhya* asserts, because something cannot evolve from nothing. There must be a root, a primary essence out of which all we can see and touch evolves. *Prakriti* is a kind of logical necessity, but not something that our senses can experience. And since it does not evolve from anything, it is eternal and indestructible.

Everything that we can see or touch or hear, on the other hand, is not eternal or indestructible. When we look around, we see that everything around us is time-bound, finite, moving, manifold, dependent on its environment, always swirling and combining with other things, and subordinate to something else. *Prakriti* itself is the opposite of these: it is eternal, infinite and pervasive, still and peaceful, one, independent, unmixed, and inferior to nothing. It is also unconscious, inanimate, insentient. This inert, limitless, stable *prakriti* is what gives rise to everything in the manifest cosmos.

Purusha is spirit, which like *prakriti* is eternal, infinite and pervasive. But unlike *prakriti*, *purusha* is conscious, awake. *Purusha* does not evolve from anything else, and nothing evolves from it. It is the witness and controller of all creation that is not limited by creation, but causes all and enjoys all. All existence is for the enjoyment of *purusha*, and *purusha* contains the promise of release, freedom and liberation.

Alone, *purusha* cannot act because it has no field of action, nothing to act upon. And *prakriti* cannot act alone because it is inanimate, unconscious. The manifestation of the universe of form depends on *purusha* and *prakriti* coming into contact with each other – they are the primal knower and known, the essential subject and object. Their coming together is, as the text says in *Kārikā* 21, like the coming together of a person who is blind and a person who is lame. They rely on each other for functions that each are incapable of on their own. And everything that we know and love and fear and crave and despise and enjoy and cringe away from depends on their union (*yoga*).

The Gunas

Every material thing in the universe, including our thoughts, beliefs and personality traits, arises out of *prakriti*, the primary material, when it comes into contact with *purusha*. When *purusha* and *prakriti* are separate, there is absolute stasis and balance. But when they join, an imbalance occurs in the three basic qualities or tendencies that underlie everything. These qualities are called the *gunas*.

The three *gunas* are qualities or constituent aspects of *prakriti*. They are not separate from *prakriti*, the way that cold and ice are not separate, or wetness and water. The word *guna* has the sense of a single strand of twine that's wound together to make a rope. Just as a rope owes its existence to each of the strands that comprise it, the manifest universe owes its existence to the collective, entwined interactions of the *gunas*. Everything that exists contains all three of the *gunas*, but in varying degrees. They are what creates the diversity of manifestation, and the constant change that characterizes the cosmos.

The names of the three *gunas* are *sattwa*, *rajas* and *tamas*. *Sattwa's* nature is like the pleasurable feeling of friendliness (*prīti*), it is light and bright, and it illuminates. *Rajas'* nature is like the unpleasant feeling of enmity or aversion (*aprīti)*; it is exciting and mobile, and it activates. Tamas' nature is like delusion or stupefaction (*vishāda*); it is heavy and enveloping, and it restrains.

Everything in creation contains all three *gunas* in varying combinations and degrees of strength. And the *gunas* themselves are interdependent: they support, hinder and produce each other. Just like a lamp is made up of a wick, fire and oil, three elements that interact through their mutual opposition to each other, the *gunas* join in interactive struggle to create everything, initiating a successive evolution of forms out of *prakriti*.

Buddhi and Ahankara

The first *tattwa* to evolve from *prakriti* is called *mahat*, which is also called *buddhi*. *Buddhi* is determination, or will, pure intentionality. It is sometimes compared to the swelling in the ocean before a wave forms. The word *mahat*, has the sense of great or vast, so this *tattwa* is essentially the vast collective desire, if we can imagine desire as a primal force without a specific attachment. It is the urge toward differentiation and variation, as the primal oneness of *prakriti* moves toward multiplicity.

Buddhi is colored by the *gunas*. When it is leaning toward *sattwa* (light), buddhi is imbued with virtue, knowledge, equanimity and power. When it leans toward *tamas* (darkness), it is infused with the opposite qualities of iniquity, ignorance, attachment and weakness.

As differentiation occurs and the one becomes many, there is a *tattwa* that crystalizes the many into individuals. This *tattwa* is called *ahankara*, or the I-maker. Ahankara is often translated as ego because it is what creates our individual sense of identity, or experience of being a self that is different, separate from our environment, unique. But we have to remember that when the *Sankhya Kārikā* was written, Freud was thousands of years away, and our current understanding of the word *ego* is overlaid with lots of concepts from modern psychology that would not have been intended or understood in the word *ahankara*. We tend to think of ego as something selfish, greedy, lustful and petty. We hear about building a healthy ego or taming the ego as if it's a circus animal or a pet. The *Sankhya Kārikā's* use of the work *ahankara* is simpler, referring to self-awareness, self-consciousness, to the force of nature that creates the experience of individuality. To what degree that individuality is colored by *sattwa*, *rajas* or *tamas* is a different matter.

It's important to remember that, at this point in the cascade of evolution initiated by the interplay of the *gunas*, there are no physical elements – no air, no fire, no water, no earth. There are no people, no embodied experiences, and no memories. There is only the essential ground of being giving way to the cosmic will to diversity, and then to a kind of force of gravity with the potential to contain individuality and provide a sense of I/me/mine to each individual form.

The Group of Eleven

Eleven more *tattwas* evolve out of *ahankara*. The first of these is *manas*, usually translated as mind. The next ten are called *indriyas*, or capacities. The first five are the powers of sense, embodied as our sense organs. These are called the *jñānendriyas*: eye (power of vision), ear (hearing), nose (smell), tongue (taste), and skin (touch). The other five *indriyas* are the capacities of action, the *karmendriyas*: the power to express, embodied as speech, the power to grasp, embodied as hands, the power to move, embodied as feet, the power to excrete, embodied as lower bowel and urinary system, and the power to procreate, embodied as the reproductive organs.

Manas is what connects and integrates the experiences and actions of the *jñānendriyas* and the *karmendriyas*. It has the added capacity of reflection, and is also sometimes grouped with *buddhi* and *ahankara* as one of the three internal organs, *antahkaranam*. The *antahkaranam* are called the gatekeepers because they apprehend all the incoming sensory information that passes through the *indriyas*, or the gates. The *antahkaranam* function in the past, present and future, while the *indriyas* function only in the present.

All of the *indriyas* are said to perform their specific functions as a result of mutual impulse. Nothing independently causes them to function per se. It is the collective action that arises together, and their collective purpose is the enjoyment of the *purusha*. As *Kārikā* 36 states, they shine like a light on all things, presenting them to *buddhi* for the sake of *purusha*. And as it is *buddhi* that facilitates the enjoyment of creation by *purusha*, it is *buddhi* that has the capacity to discern the difference between *purusha* and *prakriti*.

Tanmātras and Mahābhūtas

The *indriyas*, the powers of experience and action, require something to experience and something on and in which to act. And so *manas* also evolves the *tanmātras*, literally that which can be measured. The *tanmātras* are the subtle elements of experience: sight, sound, odor, flavor and touch. These elements are non-specific, meaning that they are not material, more like principles of matter than the actual stuff that we can see and touch.

It is out of these *tanmātras* that the physical elements, or *mahābhutas* arise. These are ether, air, fire, water and earth. Just like a painting needs to be painted on something, a canvas, a wall, etc., and as something physical is required to block the light and cast a shadow, all the elements of form, the *mahābhūtas*, require the *tanmātras*. The *tanmātras* are the canvas on which *mahābhūtas* are painted. The *mahābhūtas* are the vehicles of expression and experience for the *tanmātras*.

Mahābhutas are not actual physical substances that we can hear and touch and see and taste and smell. They are the elemental principles that underlie all substance. Everything in the universe is a modification of these five *mahābhutas*, influenced by the three gunas.

Summary

Because these fundamental elements of reality are so widely referenced in yoga-related texts, let's review the Sanskrit and English terms:

1. *Purusha* – pure spirit
2. *Prakriti*, also called Mūla-Prakriti – primal material, or root of matter
3. *Mahat* or *Buddhi* – will, determination, also sometimes called discrimination, intellect and the witness
4. *Ahankara* – the I-maker, *ego*, the force that creates the experience of subjectivity
5. *Manas* – the thinker, mind, that which integrates sensory information and organizes the powers of action
6-10. *Jñānendriyas* – powers of sense, literally capacities of knowing
6. *Śrota* – power of hearing
7. *Tvak* – power of feeling via the skin (touch)
8. *Cakshus* – power of vision
9. *Rasana* – power of taste
10. *Ghrāna* – power of smell

11-15. *Karmendriyas* – powers of action

11. *Vāk* – power of speech
12. *Pāni* – hands, the power to grasp
13. *Pāda* – feet, the power to move
14. *Upastha* – genitals, the power of procreation
15. *Pāyu* – anus, the power to digest and excrete
16-20. *Tānmatras* – that which can be measured, the subtle elements
16. *Śabda* – sound
17. *Sparśa* – touch
18. *Rūpa* – form or color
19. *Rasa* – flavor

20. *Gandha* – odor

21-25. *Mahābhūtas* – the elements, differentiated forms of the cosmic substance

21. *Ākāśa* – ether, the vacuum, the emptiness that holds the other four elements;
    - *ākāśa* can be heard, but not apprehended by the other senses
22. *Vāyu* – air, wind, motion, causes pressure
    - *vāyu* can be heard and felt, but not apprehended by the other senses
23. *Tejas* – fire, light, radiance, causes expansion
    - *tejas* can be heard, felt, and seen, but not tasted or smelled
24. *Āpas* – water, fluidity, causes contraction
    - *āpas* can be heard, felt, seen, and tasted but not smelled
25. *Prithivī* – earth, solidity, causes cohesion
    - *prithivī* can be heard, felt, seen, tasted and smelled

Sankhya Summary

Sanhkya is a way of understanding ourselves and the universe that has had a great influence on thousands of years of spiritual seeking in many different traditions. It describes a universe in which everything except the pure, infinite spirit is inert, unconscious, just being churned and shaped by the processes of nature. This includes the objects that we see, hear and touch, as well as our thoughts, emotions and beliefs. It includes our personality, what we usually experience as *I,* the *me* that we think of as having free will and choice.

In the *Sankhya* view, the ego, which we normally experience as *I*, does not have free will. It is bound by the modes of nature and subject to the flow of karma from the past that shapes our lives. On its own, it is actually not even conscious, like a piece of wood floating downstream, swirled and tossed by eddies, bouncing off of rocks, plunging over waterfalls and then surfacing again due to its natural buoyancy. The laws of the natural world shape and govern all aspects of our lives, unless and until we touch the truth of our being.

Our pure consciousness, or spirit, which is totally free and at peace, witnesses and enjoys the objects, thoughts, ideas and emotions that it touches, but it does not influence them. It experiences, but is not attached or harmed or changed at all by what it experiences. The pure spirit, the clear unadulterated consciousness becomes identified with the material ego. It is confused and deluded into thinking that the ego is what it is, and this is why we suffer. If we can understand what's really going on, who we really are, and disentangle ourselves from identification with material reality, then we can rest in the truth of our being and be free.

Chapter - 6

Patañjali's Yoga Sūtra – The Path of Purification

"Yoga is when the mind stops spinning."
— Patañjali's Yoga Sūtra (1.2)

"Yoga is samādhi."
— Vyāsa's Bhāshya (1.1)

Sometime between 5,000 BCE and 500 CE, a person who may have been named Patañjali, or maybe several people, wrote a text that may have been called the Yoga Sūtra, or perhaps the Yoga Shastra, or possibly something else. Sometime later, maybe one year, maybe five-hundred years, another person who may have been named Vyāsa, maybe the same Vyāsa who wrote the Mahābhārata and compiled the Vedas, or maybe a different Vyāsa, or possibly someone using a pseudonym (maybe Patañjali himself?), wrote a commentary that explained and gave context to the original text.

In his "biography" of the Yoga Sūtra, the Indologist David Gordon White says, "When I began this project, I was of the opinion that *classical yoga* – that is, the Yoga philosophy of the Yoga Sūtra...was in fact a tradition extending back through an unbroken line of gurus and disciples, commentators and copyists, to Patañjali himself, the author of the work who lived in the first centuries of the Common Era. However, the data I have sifted through over the past three years have forced me to conclude that this was not the case."

On the other hand, in his book "The Secret of the Yoga Sūtra", Pandit Rajmani Tigunait, PhD, writes, "Texts dating back approximately one-thousand years list seventy-one masters in the Sri Vidya tradition, beginning with the sage Kapila and ending with the eighth-century master Shankaracharya. Patañjali is fortieth on the list. The tradition has continued uninterrupted from the time this list was compiled up through the present."

TM Krishnamarcharya was arguably the founder of modern yoga. His son TKV Desikachar, developer of Viniyoga, wrote his father's biography. In it he describes his father's apprenticeship with a cave-dwelling yogi in Tibet, from whom he "not only learned Patañjali's Yoga Sūtra by heart, but he also learned to chant them with an exactness of pronunciation, tone and inflection that echoed as nearly as possible their first utterance thousands of years earlier." This statement inherently implies an unbroken line of oral transmission through which the "exactness of pronunciation, tone and inflection" would have been preserved.

And in his translation and commentary on the Yoga Sūtra, Swami Satchidananda describes specifically how the teacher Patañjali would expound "carefully coordinated Yogic thought," while "His students jotted them down in a sort of shorthand using just a few words which came to be called the Sūtras." He seems to know for sure not only that Patañjali was one individual person, but also that the sūtra form evolved from the way his students transcribed the teachings.

These excerpts represent just a few of the vast array of divergent assertions about the text that we in the modern west usually call Patañjali's Yoga Sūtra. They are the tip of a massive iceberg that includes the perspectives of classical Indian commentators, modern scholars in the western academic tradition, Indian ascetics (yogis), and members of the modern western yoga culture (who also refer to themselves as yogis). Each of these groups approaches the text with their own assumptions, agendas, and underlying beliefs about the nature of reality.

Patañjali

And while many practitioners of modern yoga appreciate Patañjali as the founder of yoga, the Indian traditions more often cite other founders like Śiva, Hiranyagarbha or Yājñavalkya. In fact descriptions of yoga's origins in the Puranas and epics never mention Patañjali. An author of the same name did write a famous commentary called the *Mahābhāshya* on the seminal Sanskrit grammar by Panini. And an author named Patañjali also wrote a great treatise on Ayurveda, the Indian medical and healing science. Whether the author of these three diverse texts was one person, two, or three remains a topic of debate among scholars, but a common view in Indian popular tradition is that Patañjali was an epic genius who elucidated Panini's grammar, compiled and expounded on healing and medicine, and founded the yoga tradition. As the tenth-century King Bhoja wrote in his commentary on the Yoga Sūtra, "He removed the impurities of mind through yoga, of speech through grammar, and of the body through medicine. I join my hands and bow to Patañjali, the best of sages."

Patañjali is the name of one of the Divine Serpents in several Puranas, and there is also a South Indian story about an incarnation of the Lord of Serpents who took human form in order to experience Śiva's grace. When his mother first held him, she was shocked to find that he was half-human and half-serpent, so she dropped him to the floor. The name Patañjali has the sense of *dropped from the hand*. During the second millennium CE, these stories about Patañjali the incarnation of the Divine Serpent seem to have been woven into a myth in which he was an incarnation of Anantaśesha, Vishnu's eternal serpent companion, who came to the Earth to enlighten humanity and alleviate suffering through the teachings of yoga. In the most common modern version of the story, Patañjali's mother was a great yogi who had prayed for a son, and a half-human and half-serpent boy was dropped (*pata*) into her hands as she held them in *anjali mudra*.

In considering Patañjali's identity, we'll need to see what line of reasoning resonates most with our own intuitive heart. Was he a half-man, half-serpent incarnation of Anantaśesha who descended to Earth for the benefit of humankind? Or was the name a pseudonym for several authors who compiled the collected wisdom of yoga? Was he a Buddhist, a practicing yogi, a scholar? There is evidence for any of these theories. But in the absence of a clear answer, what is important is that we honor the spirit of Adiyogeśvara, the original master of yoga, the Divine Force that first imparted the wisdom and promise of yoga to humankind. It may have been Patañjali, or Śiva, or Hiranyagarbha. Regardless, if we receive something from yoga, we give ourselves a great gift by opening our hearts with awe, gratitude, and bowing to its source. And when we honor the source and lineages that brought yoga to us, we cultivate humility and avoid the widespread modern western tendency to appropriate wisdom and beauty from cultures other than our birth culture without proper appreciation or acknowledgment.

Commentators Old and New

It makes sense that the 196 terse aphorisms that have come to be known as the Yoga Sūtra have been so variously understood, translated and described. They are shrouded in mystery, and their simple content leaves so much room for interpretation. The sūtras themselves are made up of almost all nouns, with some adjectives and prepositional conjunctions, and only four verbs in the entire text. Also, within the six orthodox schools of Indian spiritual philosophy, it has been common practice historically for scholars and teachers to write commentaries on texts in which they seek to make the texts relevant to their particular culture and time. It's like the way the Constitution of the United States is hashed out and re-contextualized over and over by judges and legal scholars who try to apply its basic laws to a world that is dramatically different from the one in which it was written.

Vyāsa's Bhāshya

There is one particular commentary that stands out among the rest, and some scholars even argue that it was written by Patañjali himself as a way of explaining the meaning behind the dense language of the *sūtras*. Others argue that the Yoga Sūtra was originally a Buddhist text, and this commentary was added to contextualize it within the Vedic tradition. The language of the text is more like a Sanskrit-Pali hybrid than the classical Sanskrit in which the other major ancient texts were written; the sūtra style was common among Buddhists, and many of the assertions in the Yoga Sūtra can be found in Buddhist texts.

Regardless of why it was written, the *Bhāshya*, widely appreciated as foundational commentary on the Yoga Sūtra, is ascribed to Vyāsa, which is also the name of the person who is said to have compiled the Vedas and written the Mahabharata (the 180,000+ verse epic in which we find Bhagavad Gita). Here again we run into a divergence between modern scholarship, with its adherence to the dogma of materialism, and the tradition itself, which allows for a more open and fluid understanding of reality. Many modern scholars say that the name *Vyāsa*, which has the sense of one who segments or compiles, is just a label for texts that were written by many different people. But the popular Indian tradition disagrees, honoring Vyāsa as a saint and scholar beyond compare.

There were many commentaries and discussions of the Yoga Sūtra written during the first 1300 years CE. Then it seems to have faded from view for a few hundred years, until it was introduced to the west through Vivekandanda, the Theosophists, and students of TV Krishnamacharya. These three main sources all focused primarily on the eight limbs described in the second and third pādas, giving little or no attention to the other 155+ sūtras. They also sparked a renaissance that has led to the Yoga Sūtra being required reading for any reputable yoga teacher training or in-depth study course. It is definitely curious that this text, which makes no reference at all to yoga postural practice of any kind, would be the poster text for modern western yoga culture.

The thing that Vivekananda, the Theosophists, and TV Krishnamacharya's students had in common was that they were all seeking to introduce their teachings to the western world, while at the same time tying them to an ancient source. They were innovators and evangelists; they were compelled to offer their unique form of healing and comfort to the suffering world. And perhaps they had a sense that people tend to trust the tried and true more than they trust the new. Either way, they all leaned upon the Yoga Sūtra as a way to legitimize their teachings. Patabhi Jois, TV Krishnamaharya's star student, has probably had more influence than anyone else on what we see happening in yoga studios throughout the modern western world. He called his yoga "Ashtanga Yoga," referencing the eight-limbed path of the Yoga Sūtra, even though what he specifically was teaching had very little to do with any of those limbs, and even though he seems to have run quite loosely with the first foundational limb related to moral conduct.

And he wasn't the only one. Because so many people are exposed to the Yoga Sūtra today, many of them secondhand through English translations, there is a good amount of cherry-picking going on. It's very common for people to take one or a few sūtras and define them out of context in a way that corroborates their own perspectives. Using the Yoga Sūtra to legitimize one's own approach to yoga is tempting, and to some degree hard to avoid. But we should be wary of cultural appropriation. At a certain point, using an ancient Indian text to legitimize a modern teaching in a capitalist environment without fully taking in the whole text, becoming familiar with the primary commentary, or learning to read the text in its original language, is manipulation. If we want to actually respect Patanjali's intent, to seek the authentic spirit of the Yoga Sūtra, we need to take the text as a whole, including Vyāsa's Bhāshya.

Regardless of how we got here, the Yoga Sūtra is probably the most important and widely read text in the modern western yoga culture. The ultimate aim of the text itself is stillness, silence, and separation from the material world, and yet a culture rooted in exercise and capitalist consumerism claims it as its own. It's kind of an exquisite, hopeful irony, and it does seem to have kept yoga culture from veering too far off toward a narcissistic meltdown. The Yoga Sūtra urges us to look within for the source of our being, for the truth of who we are. They ask us to dig beneath the layers of habitual identification with our surface self and seek the essence of consciousness itself, the radiant, pure, free spiritual being that illuminates this world through its eternal, untainted vision.

Samādhipāda

The text of the Yoga Sūtra is made up of four *pādas*, literally feet. The first is called *Samādhipāda*. While the word *samādhi* doesn't actually appear until sūtra 46, in his commentary on the first sūtra Vyāsa says "Yoga is *samādhi*". This is not surprising, given that the word has the sense of bringing together or joining, which is similar to the sense of the word *yoga* as union. He goes on to say that in *samādhi*, the consciousness permeates all five of its planes: raving, forgetful, oscillating, one-pointed, and self-possessed. And he specifies that when consciousness is raving, forgetful or oscillating, it doesn't stand in yoga. A one-pointed consciousness illuminates reality, destroys afflictions, loosens the bonds of karma, and brings about self-possession.

Sri Aurobindo defines *samādhi* as 'yogic trance.' He notes that "The importance of Samādhi rests upon the truth which modern knowledge is rediscovering, but which has never been lost in Indian psychology, that only a small part...of our own being comes into our ken or into our action. The rest is hidden behind in subliminal reaches of being ...The greatest value of the dream-state of Samādhi lies...in its power to open up easily higher ranges and powers of thought, emotion, will by which the soul grows in height, range, and self-mastery... Especially, withdrawing from the distraction of sensible things, it can, in a perfect power of concentrated self-seclusion, prepare itself... for access to the Divine, the supreme Self, the transcendent Truth."

Where To Begin?

Many modern teachers, in their commentaries on the Yoga Sūtra, have suggested that it's best for new students to begin with the second *pāda*, which is much more practically oriented and provides the outlines of a practice leading toward this state of *samādhi*. This makes a certain amount of sense. The practices of yoga reveal their fruits progressively, regardless of what we think about them. And in general, thinking too much about our destination doesn't get us any closer to it. Instead it can lead us to confuse abstractions with experiences, and think that because we have an intellectual understanding of *samādhi*, we have achieved it.

On the other hand, there is value in understanding the direction of our journey. *Samādhipāda* reveals great insights about the nature of the mind, why we suffer, and what happens as our consciousness becomes progressively purified. The first *pāda* sets the stage for the applications of *kriyā* yoga and the eight limbs that are described in the second *pāda*. Skipping over it would leave us with a superficial understanding of what and why we are practicing yoga at all.

Sabīja and Nirbīja Samādhi

Most of the first *pāda* builds toward the realization of what Patañjali calls *sabīja samādhi*, or *samādhi* with seeds. Vyāsa says that these seeds have come from material reality, so when they sprout they replicate the confusions and delusions inherent to material reality. Seeds may be thought of as impressions within our consciousness that sprout into ideas and assumptions. These impressions are shaped by our experiences of self and other, me and you, this and that.

Patañjali then describes how, when we stop analyzing or judging our experiences, when we stop reflecting on experience at all, our consciousness is purified and able to directly touch the field of absolute truth, or *ritambharā prajñā*. In this field of absolute truth, Vyāsa says that there is not even the faintest hint of falsehood. The impressions produced by a direct experience of the field of truth overcome all our habitual beliefs, ideas, thoughts and preferences. And when even those impressions fall away, we find ourselves in a state of seedless *nirbīja samādhi*. The mind itself, freed from its duties, falls away, and the spirit is fully established in itself, leaving us pure and liberated.

The central message of the Yoga Sūtra is tied to this state of freedom and independence. The final *sūtras* of both the third and fourth *pādas* call it *kaivalya*, which has the sense of aloneness, standing apart from all that is not real, and resting in the ultimate reality: the pure undiluted Self. The cosmology of the Yoga Sūtra is based in *Sanhkya*, which describes a universe created by the joining of *purusha*, or pure spirit, with *prakriti*, material form. Through this joining, *purusha* becomes entangled with *prakriti* and comes to falsely believe that it is *prakriti*. The path to freedom prescribed by *Sankhya* involves the *purusha* remembering its true nature, which never changed during its false identification with *prakriti*. The Yoga Sūtra takes up this theme and describes a path to the liberation of *purusha* through self-knowledge. It is a path of the purification of falsehood, a path that leads from the darkness of ignorance to the light of truth.

Yogas-Citta-Vritti-Nirodha

We begin with a definition of yoga as *citta-vritti-nirodha*. *Citta* is often translated as mind or heart-mind, but since these words have lots of baggage in current English I have chosen to use the word consciousness. *Vrittis* are the swirling whorls of thought that hypnotically draw our consciousness in and spin us around and around. You can imagine a stream where rocks create eddies, little vortices of swirling water that draw in anything that comes within their orbit. *Vrittis* are like these little eddies in our mind that distract the smooth and seamless flow of consciousness. Vyāsa alludes to the fact that producing *vrittis* is the natural work of the mind: not something that a broken mind does, but something that every mind does. So the cessation of *vrittis* implies the cessation of the mind itself.

Our understanding of *sūtra* 1.2 hinges on how we translate the word *nirodha*. Some translations lean in the direction of suppression, which gives this sūtra the spirit of willful domination. We might say that we are doing yoga when we work at stopping the mind from spinning, or that when we have suppressed our thoughts, then we have achieved a state of yoga. Other translations lean in the direction of cessation, or release, giving the *sūtra* the sense of allowing or disengagement. We might say that we're doing yoga when we allow our mind to settle, or that when we release our thoughts, we have achieved a state of yoga. This is an important distinction, because this key *sūtra* provides a definition of yoga itself, toward which the whole text is dedicated. Is yoga an act of suppression or an act of release? Various commentators have taken up both sides of this conundrum.

Once the *citta-vrittis* have been either suppressed or otherwise stilled, then the 'seer' becomes established, rooted in itself. This metaphor of the seer comes back again and again in the Yoga Sūtra. Vyāsa equates the seer with *purusha*, the pure spirit of *sankhya*, which is able to sink into the experience of its true self in the absence of mental fluctuations. Otherwise, when the mind is spinning, *purusha* tends to identify with the *vrittis*, losing its sense of self.

Abhyāsa and Vairāgya

So what to do? How do we approach this process of getting the mind to quit spinning? Patañjali's answer comes in two words: *abhyāsa* and *vairāgya*. He defines *abhyāsa* as the consistent effort to persevere over a long period of time with sincerity and attentiveness. And *vairāgya*, he says, is the mastery of our inherent thirst after things that we see, hear and touch. So regardless of how we define *nirodha*, we are reminded here that it is not easily achieved, something with which anyone who has sought to still their mind will probably agree.

Now Patañjali describes how we can move from *vritti-sarupyam* (identification with the *vrittis*) to *sabīja samādhi*. He offers that we can seek true knowledge of any object by traveling inward from a thought about it, to contemplation (sustained thinking) on it, and that sustained contemplation will give way to the joy of identification with the object of our contemplation. Or we can practice stopping thoughts as they arise. Some souls, having attained a degree of spiritual mastery in previous lives, incarnate with innate capacities that reveal themselves spontaneously, and don't need to travel the long and arduous road of practice to achieve *samādhi*. But for most of us, the profound insights that arise from *samādhi* will be supported by faith, which nurtures stamina and endurance. When our aspiration is intense, we move quickly.

Īśvara-Pranidhāna

And then Patañjali seems to offer an alternative. Specifically, he uses the word *vā*, which means *or*. We can progress toward *samādhi* through identification with an object, or by practicing stopping our thoughts, as long as our efforts are consistent and our aspiration intense. Or, says Patañjali, we can surrender everything to *īśvara*. There is considerable debate among modern commentators about who or what is meant by the word *īśvara*. The general translation in modern India is *Lord*, as in God, the Almighty. But some scholars say that at the time that the Yoga Sūtra was written, the sense of the word was not a divine being, but a guru, a teacher in the lineage of yoga. Still others argue that *īśvara* is an abstraction representing the collective wisdom of the universe. Vyāsa, however, tells us that *īśvara* is ever free, the one who manifested the scriptures, the highest unequalled Divine Lord.

What Patañjali seems to be suggesting is that a possible path to *samādhi* can be found through surrendering, praying, offering oneself and one's sense of self to what he calls *purusha-viśesha* – or "a different sort of *purusha*" that is independent of the karmic cycle, that contains the seed of all wisdom, and that is the eternal teacher of all teachers. Whether we want to view this *īśvara* as a personality like Krishna or Śiva (as some have) or an impersonal storehouse of wisdom (as others have), is less important than the emphasis Patañjali is placing on surrender. We offer ourselves to the one transcendent soul from which all knowledge flows, the one whose expression is the primordial sound *AUM*, and who we can know by chanting *AUM*. We hand over responsibility for our progress, our practice, our path to the one who knows, and we sing the name of this one, which is AUM.

Then we come to the obstacles to practice, which are the same regardless of the path that we take. Disease, apathy, doubt, carelessness, lethargy, temptation, erroneous views, ungroundedness, and regression, plus discomfort, negativity, agitation, and disturbed breathing all block our passage and tug at our heels as we traverse the path of yoga. But consistent focus will carry us through. And we can purify our consciousness, clearing out these obstacles that cling like cobwebs. We do this by remaining friendly, compassionate and equanimous in the face of pleasure or pain, virtue or vice. We can also purify our consciousness through prāṇāyāma, or by developing our sensitivity. Or we can seek to perceive the radiance that defeats all sorrow, or release attachment to pleasure. Lucid dreaming and concentrating (meditating) on anything whatsoever also support the purification process. Then the pure crystal of our consciousness more perfectly reflects reality as it is.

As our waking consciousness becomes purified, our memory also undergoes a process of purification. Objects reveal their inherent emptiness, and we recognize that all forms arise from formlessness, all sounds arise from silence, and all creation arises from emptiness. Each of these realizations characterizes *sabīja samādhi*, which as we previously discussed is the precursor to *nirbija samādhi* and *kaivalya*, ultimate liberation.

Sādhanapāda

The word *sādhana* has the sense of progressing, accomplishing. The *Sādhanapāda* is often translated as the chapter on practice. And it begins with a *sūtra* that says *tapah-svādhyāya-iśvarapranidhānāni kriyāyogah*. *Kriyā* yoga, the yoga of action, or the active yoga, consists of *tapas*, *svādhyāya* and *īśvarapranðidhāna*. We have already explored *īśvarapranidhāna*. *Tapas* is the contained heat of spiritual aspiration, and Vyāsa defines *svādhyāya* as study of the scriptures and the chanting of *AUM*. These three make up the active yoga, which has as its purpose the cultivation of *samādhi* and weakening the unhelpful states of mind (the word Patañjali uses is *kleshas*), like ignorance, egoism, clinging to pleasure, clinging to suffering, and our innate fear of death.

The Kleshas

These *kleshas* are subtle, and they arise from the storehouse of *karma* that travels with us from life to life. They determine the circumstances into which we are born, our life span, and the experiences we encounter during life. But they don't determine our happiness, which depends on how we respond to our life circumstances. No matter what occurs in our life, we choose our response. We can receive an experience of pain, poverty or loss with despair, with self-protection and armoring, with fear or with self-offering, trust and patience. We can see every challenge as an undeserved misfortune or as an opportunity for growth and deepening of self-understanding.

The unhelpful states of mind can be caught and reversed through focused concentration, which stills the spinning mind. In the stillness beyond the *vrittis*, the 'seer' disentangles itself from the 'seen' and emerges free and radiant. We can avoid future suffering by remembering that the seer only sees. It does not judge or react in any way. Even though we become confused and come to identify with that which we see (including our thoughts and personality), our essence remains pure and untroubled by this confusion.

When the ignorance that causes our confusion fades, then the process of seeing, knowing and perceiving is freed from the object of perception. We realize who is the master and what is the possession. This freedom is nourished by what Patañjali calls *viveka-khyāti*. Vyāsa describes *viveka-khyāti* as the ability to discern between the purusha and *sattva guna*. *Sattva guna* is the most light-filled, clear, peaceful quality in the material universe. When we experience the radiant tranquility of *sattva guna*, we may feel that we are experiencing the pure spirit. But *purusha* is beyond even this, and it takes a highly sensitive discernment to be able to sense the difference.

The Eight Limbs

How do we achieve this highly sensitive discernment? We achieve it by practicing the eight limbs, *ashtau-angāni*, of yoga. For many modern yogis, this is where the Yoga Sūtra begins. But we have covered a great deal of ground to get here, and all of it is useful in understanding the eight limbs and the foundation upon which they rest. Most importantly, yoga itself and the trajectory of the text from surface spinning consciousness to *nirbīja samādhi* has been defined and elaborated. And we have been given a process of active yoga to help us overcome unhelpful states of mind, which prepares us for the practices outlined in the eight limbs.

Yamas

Aligning with the general trend of Patañjali's teaching, the eight limbs progress from outer to inner. We begin with the *yamas*, or social ethics that govern our relationships to the world around us. The path of yoga is transformative, and so it involves disturbing the ego's habits and loosening its perceived grip on things. The transition from an ego-centered life to a spirit-centered life can be disorienting. These moral observances provide a contained bridge from the identification with ego to the identification with spirit. As commitments, they remind us how to act as we set out into the uncertain and unpredictable terrain of yoga.

Sri Aurobindo defines yama as "any self-discipline by which the rajasic egoism and its passions and desires in the human being are conquered and quieted into perfect cessation." Patañjali lists the yamas as:

1. *ahimsa* – non-harming; when practiced, hostility in the environment ceases
2. *satya* – truthfulness; when practiced, the results of action are sure
3. *asteya* – non-stealing; when practiced, all jewels are within reach
4. *brahmacarya* – following the path of brahman; established in it, one gains virility
5. *aparigraha* – non-hoarding; when firm in it, one gains understanding of the meaning of life

Niyamas

After the *yamas*, which describe how we should relate to the world around us, Patañjali introduces the *niyamas*, which describe how we should relate to ourselves. They are:

1. *śauca* – cleanliness; leads to disgust with our own body as well as others, leads to the purity of sattva, a happy mind, one-pointedness, victory over the senses, and readiness to witness the soul (there is a lot of argument among modern commentators about the word *jugupsā*, which is generally translated as disgust. Pandit Rajmani Tigunait provides a nuanced view. He says, "We do not clean our

house for the purpose of discovering how dirty it is so we can use this discovery to cultivate disgust for it, and, in turn, use that disgust to motivate us to abandon the house...Yet only when we begin to clean our house do we notice how pervasive and subtle the dirt is and how deeply ingrained it has become." This makes sense, but does not square with Vyāsa's commentary, which describes the yogi recognizing that the body is impure even when washed, and thus releasing attachment to it)
2. *santosha* – universal acceptance; leads to unexcelled happiness
3. *tapas* – the heat of spiritual aspiration; destroys impurities and leads to mastery over the body and sense organs (according to Vyāsa *tapas* helps us tolerate the pairs of opposites like hunger/thirst and heat/cold)
4. *svādhyāya* – self-study (according to Vyāsa study of the scriptures and chanting of AUM); leads to communion with our *ishta-devata*, the unique divine being who guides us
5. *īśvarapranidhana* – surrender to īśvara; leads to the attainment of *samādhi*

Āsana

Having covered the outer and inner observances, we are then brought further in and invited to take a seat that is steady, stable and sweet. Though Patañjali uses the word āsana, he does not describe any particular postures. Vyāsa does list thirteen postures, all of which are seated and appropriate for meditation, including *padmāsana*, *vīrāsana*, *bhadrāsana*, and *dandāsana*. Whatever posture we take, we should be able to release effort and focus our attention on the infinite so that we are not distracted by the pairs of opposites (hunger/thirst, heat/cold, sitting/standing, etc).

Prāṇāyāma and Pratyāhāra

Once we have arrived in our effortlessly stable posture, we can begin *prāṇāyāma*, or separating the inhale and exhale and bringing them to stillness. The inhale, exhale, and suspension of the breath become long and subtle. We take fewer breaths, and longer, deeper breaths. And then the breath transcends all inhale or exhale, and the covering over the eternal radiance disappears. Now the mind is ready for withdrawing the senses from their objects through *pratyahara* in preparation for beginning the inner practices of concentration and meditation.

In review, the first five limbs of yoga are:

1. *yama* – social ethics
2. *niyama* – personal observances
3. *asana* – posture
4. *prāṇāyāma* – breath control
5. *pratyahara* – withdrawal of the senses from their objects

Vibhūtipāda

The word *vibhūti* is used in various ways in ancient Sanskrit and Pali texts. The older, more foundational meaning seems to be connected to abundance and might, and then evolving during the development of the Puranas into something like splendor and glory. It has also come to refer to ashes from a sacred fire that devotees of Śiva apply to their foreheads, and in the Bhagavad Gītā Krishna uses the term ātma-vibhūti (soul-*vibhūti*) when he describes the many ways that he manifests himself in the world. Lastly, the word *vibhūti* also has the sense of occult powers, powers that we in our modern world would consider magical, like the ability to read minds, be two places at once, or levitate. It's likely that this sense of the word arose because of its use as the chapter heading for this third *pāda* of the Yoga Sūtra, which describes many such powers that a yogi might achieve in the course of their yogic journey. The *Vibhūtipāda* details the relationship between mind and matter, and ultimately the potential for mind to overcome the inherent limitations of material reality.

Samyama

In his commentary on the first sūtra of the third *pāda*, Vyāsa indicates that we are preparing to take another step forward on our journey within. He says that we have considered the five external limbs of yoga, distinguishing them from the remaining three more internal limbs. The first of the remaining three is *dhāranā*, which Patañjali defines as binding the conscious attention to one specific place. The word *dhāranā* is often translated as concentration, and Vyāsa gives us several examples of places that we might focus our concentration: the navel *chakra*, the heart-lotus, the shining part of the head, the tip of the nostrils, the tip of the tongue, or any external object.

Once *dhāranā* has been established, if we can keep our attention focused in the place of our choosing, untouched by any other distracting thoughts, we move into *dhyāna*, or meditation. And when, during meditation, the true nature of the object reveals itself directly, bypassing the thinking process entirely, we have touched *samādhi*. These three, *dhārana*, *dhyāna* and *samādhi*, are the remaining three internal limbs of the eight-limbed yoga. Patañjali calls the combined realization of these three *samyama*, a word that has the sense of total control, a complete reining in of our ordinarily fragmented consciousness. And he says that when we experience the victory of *samyama*, the brilliance of the highest wisdom dawns.

This progression from focus to meditation to absorption occurs in stages, and Vyāsa reminds us that it's not possible to jump from the beginning to the end without moving through the stages sequentially. "Yoga is reached through yoga. One who perseveres in yoga rejoices in yoga." And just as the first five limbs of yoga are external compared to the trio that make up *samyama*, *samyama* itself is external in relation to *nirbīja samādhi*. After our consciousness has fully united with the object of focus to the point where all thinking dissolves, and we touch the radiant splendor of the object's true essence, even this experience can fall away, leaving us in a state of seedless absorption. In this state, the inner tendencies that fuel mental activity are overcome by tendencies that fuel a still and settled consciousness. This is the shift to *nirodha* that the second *sūtra* of the first *pāda* defines as the essence of yoga.

Sanskāras

These tendencies are called *sanskāras* in Sanskrit. They are karmic impressions caused by our choices and action in the past, stretching back through countless lifetimes and stored in a kind of cosmic warehouse that follows us from life to life. Almost all humans, except those who have already achieved liberation in a previous life and have come back for a specific purpose, are born with *sanskāras* that fuel *citta-vrittis*. These *sanskāras* ignite mental activity in us and keep it swirling, resisting our best efforts to escape the whirlpool and achieve tranquility. But in the state of seedless absorption, new *sanskāras* are created that don't push in that direction. These new *sanskāras* create not swirling but stillness, and they progressively overcome the other *sanskāras*, until there is nothing else left to generate the swirl. This is *nirodha*, which eventually develops from a periodic experience into a smooth, consistent flow.

During this progressive yogic journey, the practice of *samyama* will reveal innate capacities that have been suppressed in us due to our immersion in the mental swirl. Patañjali lists several of these capacities, which he calls *siddhis*, and describes how each *siddhi* is produced by practicing *samyama* on a particular object or concept. We will explore just a few here:

Siddhi	Produced by Samyama on:
Understanding the language of all beings	The distinction between words, objects, and ideas
Knowledge of previous births	Direct perception of *sanskaras*
Knowledge of another's consciousness	Thoughts
Invisibility	The form of the body
Knowledge of the time of death	The momentum (speed) of karma, or omens
Strength	Friendship, compassion and delight, or the strength of an elephant
Knowledge of all realms	The sun
Knowledge of the organization of the stars	The moon
Ending of hunger and thirst	The hollow of the throat
Vision of the perfected ones who move in the space between heaven and earth	The light at the crown of the head
Complete knowledge of the nature of consciousness	The heart
A flash of illumination and supra-sensory hearing, touch, sight, taste and smell	The distinction between sattva guna and purusha

After listing these and other *siddhis*, Patañjali acknowledges that they are all obstacles for the mind absorbed in *samādhi*, while for the active mind they are accomplishments. Then he goes on to list several more *siddhis*, including the ability to enter the body of another, to project one's subtle body up out of the physical body temporarily or permanently, to shine with radiance, to hear all things, and to levitate and fly.

Next Patañjali describes how a yogi can gain mastery over the elements through *samyama* on their layers: from gross form to subtle form to composition of the gunas to purpose for existing. Mastery over the elements, as Vyāsa describes, allows the yogi to become as tiny as an atom, as weightless as a ray of light, or massive enough to touch the moon with a finger. And not only does the yogi's will become capable of creating, preserving, manipulating and destroying the elements, but the elements do not resist. The yogi can pass through stone. Water does not wet them, fire does not burn them. The air does not carry them. And the physical body becomes perfected: beautiful, graceful, strong, and as hard as a diamond.

Samyama on the layers of the sense organs, which are subtle to the elements, leads to mastery over them as well. Then the yogi can move through physical space as quickly as the mind, and gains mastery over the phenomenal world. Casting off the influences of the *tamas* and *rajas gunas* and, fully identified with *sattva guna*, the yogi realizes that even beyond the absolutely pure, light-filled *sattva*, there is another reality. That other reality is *purusha*, and the realization of this distinction between *sattva* and *purusha* provides mastery of all states of existence, and omniscience.

Finally, releasing even that state, all the seeds are destroyed and the yogi finds *kaivalya*, total liberation. Here Patañjali provides a warning: be wary of temptation by the devas, who may intervene with flattery and invitations to join them in their celestial abode, free from suffering. Stay fixed upon the goal of dissolving the mind. As Vyāsa says, the yogi who becomes proud will not understand that they are caught by the hair of Death.

Kaivalhyapāda

Several copies, translations and commentaries of the Yoga Sūtra from the first millennium CE had only the first three *pādas*. So some scholars speculate that *pāda* four was a later edition. One possible scenario is that the original three *pādas* were written by Buddhists, and Vyāsa's commentary and the fourth *pāda* were added to integrate the Yoga Sūtra into the Vedic philosophical framework. Like so much about the original of the Yoga Sūtra and Patañjali himself, this remains a mystery.

Kaivalyapāda doesn't introduce many new ideas, but goes back over some important lines that trace through the Yoga Sūtra, adding depth and color and subtlety, further illuminating the path toward a grand crescendo of ultimate freedom. We begin with the assertion that *siddhis* are a natural phenomenon. They arise naturally as a result of spiritual progress during previous lifetimes, through the use of herbs and elixirs, by chanting mantras, from the focused heat of spiritual aspiration, and/or from samādhi. When the forces of nature build up within a container like the human body/mind system, just like water in a glass, eventually they will overflow and manifest a transformation. The practice of yoga is a way of removing the resistance to the natural flow of forces, similar to the way a farmer simply removes obstacles to the flow of water to irrigate the fields.

When the forces of nature flow into the container of ego, or *I-ness*, consciousness becomes individuated, and individual beings act in ways that produce *karma* that's either negative, positive, or neutral. This *karma* gives rise to *sanskāras*, which merge with our inborn desire to live, and creates our unique character traits, likes, dislikes, and beliefs about reality. A mind fixed in meditation does not produce *karma*, and so the actions of a yogi in meditation are neither right nor wrong, bad or good, karmically positive or negative.

Seen By The Seer

Patañjali then goes on to describe how the one single substance that is the foundation of the creative universe gives rise to unique objects. The three *gunas* merge with our perception, which is influenced by conditioning to shape objects out of the original substance. Our conscious awareness is produced the same way. It is not self-luminous like the *purusha*, which Patañjali also calls the seer. Our conscious awareness is seen by the seer, and it comes into being through this seeing.

This may seem obscure, but it's fairly simple. Our essential individual self, that within us that sees and hears and reflects, exists because we are projected into existence by the pure undying spirit that stands behind the veil of the material universe. This spirit sees us into existence. And that pure undying spirit also sees the manifest world through us. It, being changeless, notices the changes in and around us. So we, the surface personality self that we usually experience and identify as *self*, are both seen by the seer and the vehicle of the seer's seeing the world.

And when we experience the difference between the clarity of our own seeing and the purity of the one who sees through us, this distinction between self and seer disappears. This discernment draws us toward *kaivalya*, the state of liberation that depends on nothing. Along the way, thoughts and mental/emotional impressions arise in us as a result of old *sanskāras* bearing fruit. They can be sticky, and have a tendency to pull us into identification with them. But we can send them back to where they came from.

And when we release attachment to even the higher state of consciousness that we've attained, a state that Patañjali call *dharma-megha-samādhi* arises. We are immersed in the cloud of virtue, the cloud of righteousness, and the rains of goodness pour down upon us spontaneously. All *karmas* and obstacles are washed away by this rain of grace. We are cleansed of all impurities and the changes caused by the *gunas* resolve. In the wake of these changes, we understand the inherent reason for change itself. The resolution of the *gunas* leaves us standing, free and alone, rooted in our true, brilliant nature for evermore.

Summary

Its origins are shrouded in mystery. It has been appropriated and used to give modern teachings an ancient pedigree. It was virtually unknown for hundreds of years until Swami Vivekananda and others sparked a renaissance that has steadily blossomed in the last 125 years. And the Yoga Sutra offers a concise and brilliant description of the workings of human consciousness and its aspiration toward freedom.

Taken with Vyāsa's commentary, Patañjali's exposition on yoga takes us from the swirling of the surface mind deeper and deeper within, from the unhelpful states of mind that create our suffering to greater and greater clarity. Through consistent practice and mastery over our distracting cravings, or through surrender to the Divine Lord of Creation, we gradually move toward stillness and release the impurities that cloud our perception of reality. Finally, we are able to discern our true, pure nature as eternal, deathless, and absolutely free.

The Yoga Sutra does not mention the collective movement of evolution that draws all of humanity toward this state. And it does not describe how one who has achieved liberation might live and engage with the world. It focuses on the individual path and how to stay on it in the midst of a world that lumbers slowly and grudgingly toward freedom, zigging and zagging interminably. It offers timeless guidance, inspiration, and warnings for the traveler who has chosen not to wait for the world, but to take up the path toward their own self-realization.

Today, the modern householder yogi may not have the time and space to realistically follow Patañjali's path step-by-step. The path may seem impossibly steep, unrealistically arduous. But the wisdom that the Yoga Sutra offers can reinforce our understanding of ourselves, and illuminate our own entanglements and habits that obscure our vision. It offers perennial wisdom and ageless truths, for which we can offer bows of gratitude.

Chapter - 7

Bhagavad Gītā – The Great Synthesis

I stepped through the metal detector and gave my bag to the guard, surprised by the tight security. There were cameras in the trees and military police carrying sizable guns. I asked the guard, and he explained that on the other side of the temple was a mosque, and unresolved territorial disputes contained an underlying sectarian tension. India, the land of multiplicity, of many voices crying to the divine in their own language, with their own words and rhythms, has long wrestled with how to honor this diversity and protect its people from religious fanatics.

Winding through passageways and heading down, lower and lower, I eventually reached a kind of man-made cave. Entering through one side I saw a beautiful shrine honoring the birthplace of Krishna. I was in the jail cell where his mother Devaki gave birth to him, and where her cousin Kamsa killed the seven babies born before him. When Krishna was born, the gates of the prison cell opened and the guards fell asleep, allowing his father Vasudeva to escape and carry him to the countryside and place him in the care of a farmer's wife named Yaśodā.

The atmosphere was somber and sacred. I bowed and offered my heart, and then moved through the room and out the door at the opposite end. Eventually I found my way up to the giant Bhagavata

Bhavan, a temple commemorating the *Srīmad Bhagavatam* that recounts the tales and legends of Krishna's life. This temple is several stories above the jailroom shrine, and at its front stand two giant statues of Krishna and Rādha. The room was full of worshippers singing, praying, laying themselves prostrate on the floor, weeping, and meditating. I stared at the statue, and I felt clearly that these were no stone idols. These were living presences, radiating their grace and love to all who came to honor them. I felt tears on my face, and my heart melted, opening itself to the pain and beauty of the world, carried in the hearts of these devotees who had come to bask in the loving grace of their Divine Beloveds.

Krishna the hero of *Srīmad Bhagavatam* is the Lord of Love. He embodies the love of a child for his mother, and awakens in Yaśoda the divine love of mother for son. He embodies the love shared between friends, the love of young lovers, the shared love of a community. His life is a demonstrative teaching on how to love, how to be love in all circumstances and at all times. This is the pretext for Krishna the teacher of the Bhagavad Gītā. This is the fountain from which his teaching flows.

A Practical Battlefield Discourse

The *Vedas* and the *Upanishads* cloak their wisdom in poetry and symbol. The *Rāmāyana* encloses profound spiritual truths in story, embodying its teaching in the inner and outer experiences of its characters. The *Bhagavad Gītā* wears no veil. In this "Divine Song," Krishna imparts his teaching directly to Arjuna. Krishna speaks, leading Arjuna into a progressively deeper understanding of the nature of reality and his place in it. Arjuna asks clarifying questions, expresses his doubts, gradually assimilates the teaching with Krishna's loving encouragement. This is not a lofty philosophical discourse, but a practical teaching that is meant to influence Arjuna's daily life.

> "The central interest of the Gītā's philosophy and Yoga is its attempt...to reconcile and even effect a kind of unity between the inner spiritual truth in its most absolute and integral realization and the outer actualities of our life and action." - Sri Aurobindo
>
> Essays on the Gītā

This conversation takes place on a battlefield, in the moments before the battle begins. Immense legions have massed on either side, preparing to engage. Krishna delivers his teaching in a context that could not be more urgent and dire, and this sharpens his message like the tip of a spear. Arjuna faces his own death, and the death of his friends, teachers and family.

According to the traditional cosmology, the *Bhārat* War took place in 3102 BCE, but modern scholars tend to prefer dates between 1500 and 800 BCE. The great epic poem called Mahābhārata, over 100,000 verses in length, describes the events leading up to the war, as well as depicting the war itself in great detail. The *Bhagavad Gītā* appears within the *Mahābhārata*, just seven-hundred verses in length. But the potency of its message has earned it the title of the Fifth Veda by many yogis and philosophers.

Arjuna is a great warrior, one of five *Pāndava* princes, protagonists in the *Mahābhārata*. Their cousins, the ruthless and conniving *Kauravas*, have cheated them out of their share of the kingdom, and govern the people unfairly, promoting greed and chaos. The *Pāndavas* resolve to fight the *Kauravas* to restore order and justice to the land. Arjuna is a *kshatriya*, or warrior, and his appointed role within the broader society is to protect the innocent, uphold justice, and establish order and equality. If he walks away from this duty, injustice and inequality will reign and the innocent will be preyed upon by the greedy *Kauravas*.

Purushottama

Krishna is Arjuna's charioteer, but as we discover during his teaching, he is also a direct embodiment of the Divine One. He is an *avatāra*:

> "Though I am the unborn, the imperishable, the self-existent, though I am the Lord of all existences, yet I stand upon my own Nature and come into birth by my self-Maya. Whenever there is a fading of Truth and an uprising of unrighteousness, then I loose myself into birth." (4.6, 7)
> "Neither the celestial beings nor the great sages know My birth. I am altogether and in every way the origin of the celestial beings and the great sages. Whoever knows me as the Unborn, the mighty Lord of the worlds and peoples, lives unbewildered among mortals and is delivered from all sin and evil." (10.2, 3)

Krishna is a prominent character in the *Mahābhārata*, and his divinity is hinted at throughout the text. But only in the *Gītā* is his divine identity fully revealed. He identifies himself not just as a divine being, but as the One from Whom the entire universe emerges and into Whom it returns, the One that unifies Being and Non-being. And the entire eleventh chapter describes the vision that Krishna allows Arjuna of his primordial Divine form.

Krishna's identity as the *purūshottama* (Supreme Soul) is critical to his teaching, because the axis of the teaching is love:

> "Steep your mind in Me, become My lover and adorer, become a sacrifice to Me, bow yourself to Me, and you will come to Me; this is My pledge and promise to you, for you are dear to Me. Abandon all Dhārmas and take refuge in Me alone." (18.65, 66)

Krishna not only teaches Arjuna about the nature of the universe and how to live in it, but he embodies the divine love that flows through the teaching. This is no mere theoretical philosophy, but a promise directly from the Heart of the Universe that if we surrender our smallness, our selfishness, our pettiness, our fear, if we offer every action and the fruit of every action to the Divine One, then we will be gathered into the holy arms of Divinity.

The promise of the *Gītā* is the promise of a Life Divine on Earth, in community, in action, in work and rest and play. We don't need to retreat to a cave to find peace and perfection; we can find it here in our everyday life, in the midst of fulfilling our unique individual *dharma*. We don't need to die to find Heavenly perfection and bliss; we can find it here by sacrificing everything to the One Who is Bliss and Perfection, Who is not far away in another dimension, but within us, around us, everywhere.

Krishna is the *avatāra* descended to Earth *"for the deliverance of the good, for the destruction of the evil-doers, for the enthroning of the Right, the Dharma..."* (4.8) He is also the essence of everything in the universe, including ourselves:

> *"Just as air dwells within ether, all existences dwell in Me..."* (9.6) *"And whatever is the seed of all existences, that also am I, O Arjuna; no being is there, moving or unmoving, that could be there without Me."* (10.39)

Arjuna

Throughout his life Arjuna has considered Krishna his friend. He honors Krishna's deep wisdom, but does not know his true identity. And it's with this limited consciousness that he asks Krishna to drive him out into the center of the battlefield, into the no-man's-land between the two armies that are massed on either side. Krishna steers the chariot into view of the enemy lines, and as Arjuna gazes upon the faces that he knows so well, uncles and teachers and friends, despair overtakes him.

> "Even if these, with their consciousness clouded by greed, do not see any guilt in the destruction of the family and no crime in hostility to friends, why should not we have the wisdom to draw back from such a sin, we who see, O Janārdanā (Krishna), the evil...?" (1.38-39) "It is better that the armed sons of Dhritarashtra should slay me unarmed and unresisting in the battle." (1.46)

This is a great spiritual treatise, and so one might assume that Krishna would agree with Arjuna, understanding his pain and supporting his moral disgust in the face of so terrible a work. But he does not:

> "Yield not to impotence, O Pārtha (Arjuna); it its not worthy of you. Shake off this faint-heartedness and arise!" (2.3)

Synthesis

So begins Krishna's teaching, which expands over the course of seventeen chapters and reconciles ancient and fundamental arguments about cosmology, liberation and life. Is it better to engage in action or renounce action? Is it better to seek liberation through service (*karma*), knowledge (*jñāna*), or love (*bhakti*)? Is it better to perform Vedic sacrificial rituals or perform austerities? How can we escape from suffering, what is the way to liberation?

At the time of the *Gītā's* compilation, these specific lines of inquiry were prevalent, and various schools of thought had coalesced around different perspectives. And even though the message of the *Gītā* is always a synthesis, always *yes and* rather than *either or*, these arguments have persisted and schools and sects continue to cherry-pick verses from the *Gītā* that seem to support their perspective to the exclusion of others.

But Krishna does not take sides. He weaves together a comprehensive teaching that dissolves the boundaries between arguments. He integrates them, synthesizes them, and shows that it is in their opposition that they fail, but not in their unity. He also shows that the whole is more than the sum of its parts: when we perform action and renounce the fruit of the action, when we seek liberation through service and knowledge and love, when we place our egoistic desires in the sacrificial fire and seek equanimity, and when we do all this in partnership with Him, the Holy One, then we find a peace and liberation that transcends the ways of the world but does not leave it behind.

Starting from the exhortation to stand and fight, to fulfill his *dharma*, Krishna leads Arjuna on a journey from an outer perspective to an inner perspective. Arjuna despairs over the lives that will be lost during the coming war. Krishna responds by explaining that every living being is first and foremost a soul, an infinite and immortal divine being that wears a body and personality like we wear our clothes:

> *"The embodied soul casts away old and takes up new bodies as a person changes worn-out clothes for new...It is uncleavable, incombustible, it can neither be soaked nor dried. Eternally stable, immobile, all-pervading, it is for ever and ever." (2.22, 24)*

Krishna teaches us that all beings, including ourselves, are essentially eternal. From an outer perspective, we die. But when we come to know our true selves experientially, we find that we do not die, but only transform. This differentiation between outer and inner perspective continues throughout the dialogue, and leads to the teaching that all outer laws, all outer perspectives, all reasoning and justification based solely on a vision of the outer reality are limited and incomplete. We must discover our inner selves to see truth and experience reality as it is.

> *"To break out of ego and personal mind and see everything in the wideness of the self and spirit, to know God and adore Him in his integral truth and in all his aspects, to surrender all oneself to the transcendent Soul of nature and existence, to possess and be possessed by the Divine consciousness, to be one with the One in universality of love and delight and will and knowledge, one in Him with all beings, to do works as an adoration and a sacrifice on the divine foundation of a world in which all is God and in the divine status of a liberated spirit, is the sense of the Gītā's Yoga."*
>
> - Sri Aurobindo Essays on the Gītā

Action and Inaction

One of the primary inquiries that Krishna addresses involves the relationship between spirituality and action. Many spiritual philosophies throughout time have argued that, to become free, we must leave behind the world, which is an illusion, and seek the eternal truth in stillness and silence. The Eternal, they argue, is unchanging, and all movement, all sound, all action is change. To touch the unchanging we must be unchanging ourselves. Every time we act we incur karma, which furthers our entanglements and frustrates our efforts toward freedom. But Krishna disputes this:

> *"Not by abstaining from work do we experience actionlessness, nor by renouncing work do we attain perfection. For none stand even for a moment not doing work; everyone is made to do action helplessly by Nature itself."* (3.4, 5)

Krishna reminds us that we cannot actually escape action. The heart beats, the breath flows, the mind thinks – this is part of being alive. We are subject to the fluctuations of the natural world that we inhabit. We shouldn't delude ourselves into thinking that we can escape from action and its entanglements.

Krishna's teaching has great nuance: we should continue to act, to work, but we should not be confused about who is acting:

> *"When the actions are being done by the modes of Nature, we are bewildered by egoism if we think that it is 'I' that is doing them...All beings follow their nature, and what can we do about it? Even those who know the truth act according to their own nature." (3.29, 33)*

The *modes of Nature* to which Krishna refers are the *gūnas*, the fundamental qualities of existence that make up all of manifestation. Most schools of yoga philosophy rest upon an understanding that the manifest universe is made up of three primary modes, or qualities: *tamas* (inertia, sluggishness, death, decay, heaviness, darkness), *rajas* (fire, effort, growth, activity, expansion), and *sattva* (balance, light, peace, stability). When these three *gūnas* come into complete balance, existence ceases. Every manifest being and substance arises from an imbalance in the *gūnas*.

> *"Sattva, rajas, and tamas, these gūnas born of prakriti, bind down the imperishable soul in the physical body." (14.5)*

One of the traditional schools of yoga that Krishna specifically mentions is called *Sankhya*. *Sankhya* philosophy distinguished *prakriti*, or the manifest universe, from *purusha*, or the eternal unchanging soul. Sankhya enumerated the specific *tattwas*, or basic elements of creation that are subject to and influenced by fluctuations in the *gūnas* caused by *karma*, and advised seeking and connecting to the immortal purusha as a way of escaping these fluctuations, which cause suffering. Krishna's teaching builds upon the *Sankhya* model, and agrees that understanding the *tattwas*, how they relate to each other, and the nature of their subjection to the *gūnas* is fundamental to understanding reality as it is.

Specifically, *Sankhya* teaches that, while material form and soul are distinct, mind and body are both aspects of prakriti, and thus not inherently free. Krishna teaches us that most of the time, when we think *I* am doing something, it is really the *gūnas* that are forcing action to happen. We think of ourselves as having 'free will,' but mostly we are not free, but reacting to stimulus from outside, carrying ideas we have taken in from others, fulfilling our *karma*. If we look closely at our actions and what motivates them, we begin to see a determinism shaping our beliefs, thoughts and actions that usually hides in the folds of unconsciousness.

Actually, if you google "Free will is an illusion," you'll see arguments from scientists and modern philosophers saying essentially the same thing. But what they don't say, which Krishna does, is that we do have one choice that can change the whole game. This choice is to discover and embody our deepest and truest self, which naturally receives and radiates endless love.

Equanimity

Krishna encourages us to act, but not to cling to the fruit of our actions. When we act, instead of worrying about what will happen as a result of our actions, grasping after the potential gains or trying to dodge to potential losses, we should *"Make grief and happiness, loss and gain, victory and defeat equal to thy soul..."* (2.38).

Samata, meaning equality or equanimity, is essential to perceiving one's *dhārma*. As humans, we are full of cravings and aversions. These impulses pull us in every direction, and drive our actions. They become our charioteers, taking us on chase after chase in pursuit of satisfaction. But we don't ever arrive at satisfaction, only a momentary lull of desire, which flares up again and again. For Krishna to become our divine charioteer, we must have some mastery over these impulses.

Once we stabilize this equanimity within ourselves, then we can choose to offer our motivations, our actions, and the fruits of our actions to the One Divine. When we act for the One and in the One, then we become entirely free, as the One is our true self, our true nature.

> "He who loves and strives after Me with an undeviating Yoga of devotion, he passes beyond the three *gūnas* and is prepared for joining with the One. I am the foundation of the Oneness and of immortality and of the eternal *dhārma* and of an utter bliss of happiness." (14.26, 27)

When we act as a separate self in competition with the world around us, when we grab and hoard and delude ourselves and others, then we are bound, unfree. But when we discover our true self which is unified with all, and surrender the sense of separation, when we allow the Oneness to move through us and bless the world through our action, then we are truly free. This offering of our actions and the fruits of our actions is, Krishna says, the essence of the sacrifice expounded by the *Vedas*.

We can find liberation without retreating from the world. We can align ourselves with the Supreme Heart of All Creation, letting action move through us that serves the whole, and thus truly fulfill our *svadhārma*, or unique individual *dhārma*, and act according to our *svabhāva*, or unique individual nature. We are each created as unique manifestations of the One with unique work that is indispensable to the collective evolution. The One remembers Itself as the One through us, through our love, our offering, our sacrifice.

Krishna offers a graded approach to this state of freedom. First, we must realize what's going on, recognize the situation as it is. Then we can offer our actions and their fruits to Him, the Lord and Indwelling Essence of All. Eventually, Krishna will gather us to Him and begin to direct our actions, dissolving the separation and joining us with All. But even then, in the state of yoga, or union, action does not cease. Even Krishna himself incarnates from age to age and continues to work in this evolutionary world to further the progression of the collective yoga.

Service, Knowledge, and Love

A second major synthesis that Krishna offers is that of three approaches to liberation that have historically tended to become isolated within various lineages or schools. There are those who preach a doctrine of **karma yoga** (the yoga of service), others who practice *jñāna* **yoga** (the yoga of knowledge), and others still who pursue **bhakti yoga** (the yoga of devotion). In a masterful way that gathers all the little strands of each path, Krishna weaves them together into a single teaching that encompasses and exceeds them all. And he also expands and clarifies each path, drawing out its nuances and defining it in a way that compliments the others rather than excluding them.

It is true that individuals tend to have a preference for one approach over the others, and there is nothing wrong with that. We each have our own *svabhāva*, our own unique nature. But when we say "I'm a *bhakta*," or "I'm not a *bhakta*, I'm a *jñāna*," we do run the risk of cutting ourselves off from an important aspect of ourselves. Just like the three *gūnas* exist in different proportions in every aspect of existence, the three paths of yoga exist in different proportions in all of us, and this is not static. One path may predominate for a time, giving way to the emergence of another. I may be inclined for a while toward textual study and mental inquiry in the search for myself, and then later the flame of devotion may arise within. Inevitably, as we move forward along a path of self-discovery, we will be inclined to explore different approaches to truth. If we maintain a fixed idea that one approach is ours for all time, then we will limit the soul's natural movement to freely explore all dimensions of our inner landscape.

First Krishna reconciles knowledge and service. His teaching essentially is that, when we know the nature of reality, when we have inquired into and explored the layers and phenomena of existence and come to understand the nature of causation, the reality of *karma*, and the delusion of what we normally consider free will, then our actions do not bind us:

> "As a fire kindled turns to ashes its fuel, O Arjuna, so the fire of knowledge turns all works to ashes." (4.37)

When we act from within ego-created delusion, thinking that we are an individual self that acts upon an inert and separate world, then we are unwittingly bound by the invisible consequences of our actions. But when we act from an enlightened alignment with the true self, the purusha that is inherently joined with all and thus always seeks to serve all, then our actions facilitate liberation for ourselves and others.

Krishna explains to Arjuna that he has two different aspects: a lower aspect that manifests as prakriti, and a higher aspect that is free and independent of *prakriti*:

> "Earth, water, fire, air, ether, sense-mind, ego, and reasoning mind – this is my eightfold nature. This is the lower. Know too, O mighty-armed, my other Nature which is different from this, the Supreme which becomes the individual soul and by which this world is upheld. Know this to be the womb of all beings. I am the birth of the whole world and also its dissolution." (7.4, 5, 6)

Next, Krishna joins knowledge and devotion. Truly, when we come to know the Divine One, then we cannot help but fall to our knees in devotion. And when we love the Supreme Being with all our heart, then we cannot help but come to know and understand That One. Whichever path we begin upon, we will eventually find the other, for they inevitably join.

> "At the end of many births, the seeker of knowledge attains to Me and sees that Vasudeva, the omnipresent Being, is all that is." (7.19)

This interwoven yoga of service, knowledge and devotion is Krishna's offering to Arjuna, and to the world. He invites us to find and experience all the dimensions of our relationship with the Divine, to let them flow into each other and expand each other. And when we join heart, mind and hands, unifying our life in a single direction, we are sure to arrive at our destination.

> "Devoting all thyself to Me, giving up in thy conscious mind all thy actions into Me, resorting to Yoga of the will and intelligence, be always one in heart and consciousness with Me. By aligning your heart and consciousness with Me at all times, by My grace you will pass safely through all difficult and perilous passages." (18.57, 58)

Surrender

This kind of surrender requires a shift from our usual outer perspective to an inner one. We must turn away from the outer rules, the fear of being disliked or disapproved of, the tendency to be overly concerned with others' beliefs about us and about the world. We have to leave this behind, but not in favor of the ego's desires or animal cravings that inhabit our bodies and minds. Transcending desire and egoism, we must turn to the Divine One for guidance and direction, we must lift ourselves up and offer ourselves to That One who loves us eternally and unconditionally, and Who seeks always to bring us forward in our unique work that serves simultaneously our own growth and the growth of the world toward wholeness and harmony. We must abandon an outer idea of *dhārma*, or duty, and discover our inner duty, our inner purpose for existence, and devote ourselves entirely to that.

There are structures in the world created to maintain order, to keep the pack together. When we begin to ignore these outer forms and march to our inner beat, these structures will naturally seek to bring us back into line, restricting our freedom. We may be ridiculed or threatened if we don't comply with social conventions. We may be seen as starry-eyed, idealistic, deluded, unreasonable, or unkind. These outer challenges to our freedom have to be overcome, not by the force of ego and self-will, but by an increasing surrender of our will to the force of love.

Krishna ends by asking Arjuna if his delusion has been destroyed, and Arjuna answers that, through Krishna's grace, he has regained his memory:

> *"I stand firm with my doubts dispelled. I will act according to Thy word."* (18.73)

Arjuna has determined to go to war against the *Kauravas*, and fight with nobility and courage. It is important to remember that Arjuna is a warrior, and his *svadharma* leads him into battle. Most of us will not find ourselves in a similar situation. We will not be asked to kill in the name of justice and righteousness. But we may feel the same kind of fear and repulsion to embodying the *dharma* that we have been given.

We may find as we seek our path that there are moments when what we are asked to do feels overwhelming. The Divine One tends to push our boundaries, to bring us into uncertain terrain where we can't see what is right or how to act. In the process of upsetting the ego's delusion of control, our self-concept must be transformed, and this involves facing fear and despair. When we stand there facing the impossible, sure that we will fail, and unsure if we even want to succeed, when doubts cloud our vision and fear assails us, we can remember that we are not alone. Krishna is there, ready to drive the chariot, to lead us into the fray.

The *Bhagavad Gītā* is a profound, multidimensional and beautiful work with universal implications. It transcends religion, philosophy, nationality, and time. It offers teachings that are just as relevant to us today in the twenty-first-century western world as they were thousands of years ago in Asia. This chapter has only touched upon the depth and diversity of Krishna's message, attempting to give a feeling for what he offers and its possible practical application. There is so much more, and the text is so dense and packed with wisdom that only by reading it through can you experience its fullness.

Not only that, but the *Bhagavad Gītā* is a song. It has rhythm and melody, and these are nearly impossible to carry through a translation into English. The only way to experience the amazing lyricality of the *Gītā* is to hear it sung. And more beautiful still is learning to chant the original Sanskrit, feeling the cadence and the texture of the words, the ebb and flow of emphasis and accent. Experiencing the *Gītā* becomes a spiritual practice in itself, including reading translations to understand, listening to recordings, and chanting along. It's through this kind of engagement that the *Gītā* reveals its treasure trove of mysteries and wisdom.

> *"The supreme law of action is therefore to find out the truth of your own highest and inmost existence and live in it and not to follow any outer standard or Dhārma...Offer, first, all your actions as a sacrifice to the Highest and the One in you and to the Highest and One in the world; then deliver all you are and do into his hands for the supreme and universal Spirit to do through you his own will and works in the world."*
>
> \- Sri Aurobindo Essays on the *Gītā*

Chapter - 8

The Devīmāhātmya – Glory of the Divine Mother

At the top of *Cāmundā* Hill, a half hour's drive from Indore in Central India, is a series of caves. They hold statues and shrines to various manifestations of the Divine Being, and they look like they were probably prime real estate for yogis in ancient times. Today there is a broad walkway leading from the parking lot below to the final large cave at the top, the cave inhabited by *Cāmundā* herself.

I stood outside the cave and admired the massive image of *Devi Cāmundā* painted onto the overhanging bulge of rock in the back of the cave. I looked around at the other small shrines, a Śiva *linga*, a small fire pit for *yajña* ceremonies, and a view of the plains below. And then I sat to meditate just outside the cave. As I was settling, the pujari inside the cave motioned to me to come inside. I entered, and he pointed to a little nook just to the side of the entrance, a space large enough for me to sit.

I looked up at *Cāmundā*. I closed my eyes, and she was still there. Her gleaming silver sword raised above her head, she smiled, ready to decapitate the ego and release the soul from bondage. I felt the warmth of her presence, her breath on my cheek.

I heard someone enter the cave on my left, and opened my eyes. A devotee kneeled down and placed his forehead on the cave floor below *Cāmundā*. Poised for the strike her sword flashed above his head. The poignancy of the scene overwhelmed me and tears flowed from my eyes. My hair stood on end. The devotee offered his head to the *Devī's* sword, he laid down his life before her, inviting her to do with him what she would. The Fierce Mother smiled at her beloved child, and radiant love poured from her into him, filling the cave. The name Ma, Ma, Ma, Ma filled me, overtaking all thought and infusing every inch of my being.

The Mother of All

> "I am the Lord and the Cosmic Soul; I am myself the Cosmic Body...I am the sun and the stars, and I am the Lord of the stars...I am the evildoer and the wicked deed; I am the righteous person and the virtuous deed. I am certainly female and male, and asexual as well. And whatever thing, anywhere, you see or hear, that entire thing I pervade, ever abiding inside and outside. There is nothing at all, moving or unmoving, that is devoid of me."
>
> (from The Devī Gītā, translation by C. Mackenzie Brown)

The Divine Mother is the universal aspect of the One. She pervades all existence: the universe is her body, and she lives within the heart of every being. She manifests as time and space, and every substance, action, thought, and experience is part of her. Nothing is outside her, nothing is devoid of her presence.

The Mother is matter, life and mind. As space, she stretches out her body as the field for the Oneness to experience itself in form. As time, she unfurls moment after moment, adding her holy breath to spur the process of evolution and growth toward wholeness. She is our inclination to care for each other, to honor the seamless weave that unites all. When we feed the hungry, offer hope to the hopeless, and in any way give of ourselves to nourish others, we honor her being and praise her name.

Embodiment practices like yoga asanas, qigong, walking meditation or dancing allow us to directly touch the Divine Mother. As we draw our awareness into the field of matter and flowing energy that is the human body, we can feel Her embrace as space and time. Our asana and meditation practices can be adventures of discovery, seeking and revealing Her miraculous, intricate beauty that is the fabric of all existence.

She is the very life that animates us, and She is every thought, every hope, every ache. The deepest longings of our hearts to be seen, to be whole and fulfilled are Her longings, and She is the source of all comfort, assurance, and satisfaction. We inhabit Her, and She inhabits us.

The Mother has been praised by humans forever. Ancient artwork depicting the Mother and honoring Her fertility, Her governance of the cycles of nature, and Her protection of the vulnerable has appeared throughout the world, including in the Indus Valley in northwestern India, an area that became the cradle of the Vedic culture. And there is a clear continuity between the faces and attributes of the Mother that appear in these ancient artifacts and the faces and attributes of the Mother that appear in the early yogic texts.

Divine Mother in the Rig Veda

The Divine Mother has many names and faces in the yogic tradition. In the *Rig Veda*, Aditi (a name which means *unbound*) is the mother of the devas and the twelve beings that form the Vedic zodiac, from whom the stars and planets are born. "She is the Supreme Light and all radiances proceed from her." (Sri Aurobindo). She is self-luminous, the Light that is Mother of all things, and manifests also as Usha, the divine dawn who brings with every new day more truth to the evolving Earth.

In another Vedic hymn (*Rig Veda 10.125.3-8*), the rishi speaks as the Divine Mother embodied as Vak, the primordial voice. This verse is commonly known as the *Vak Suktam* or the *Devī Suktam*:

> "I am the Queen, the gatherer-up of treasures, most thoughtful, first of those who merit worship. The devas have dispersed me and established me in many places, causing me to pervade everything.
>
> One who eats food, who sees, who breathes, who hears the spoken word does so through me alone. Even the non-perceivers of you dwell near me. Hear me if you are capable! I speak to you the truth.
>
> I speak these words myself, which are praised by both devas and humans: whomever I wish, I make them powerful, well-versed in knowledge, a sage and a wise one.
> I bend the bow for Rudra [Shiva], that his arrow may strike, and slay the hater of devotion. I rouse and order battle for the people, I created Earth and Heaven and reside as their Inner Controller.
>
> On the world's summit, I bring forth sky the Father: my home is in the waters, in the ocean as Mother. Thence I pervade all existing creatures, as their Inner Supreme Self, and manifest them with my body.

I created all worlds at my will, without any higher being, and permeate and dwell within them. The eternal and infinite consciousness is I, it is my greatness dwelling in everything."

(Translation modified from original by Ralph T.H. Griffith)

Shaktism

The *Devī Suktam* is one of the primary textual references for the tradition of Shaktism. Contrary to popular belief, most yogic ancient traditions are not polytheistic, but either monotheistic or monistic. Three major theistic lineages have emerged within the broad yogic framework. Each reveres one particular deity as the Supreme out of Whom all has emerged, Who governs and animates all, and into Whom all dissolves. All other deities are considered emanations of the One.

Vaishnavism honors Vishnu as the Supreme, Śaivism honors Śiva, and Shaktism honors Śaktī, also called Devī. These traditions have ancient roots, and have gone through various phases of development and revival over thousands of years. They all formally trace their roots to the *Vedas* and *Upanishads*, and consider the Vedic corpus to be the ultimate scriptural authority, though there are tantric sub-sects within each that deviate from this.

Aside from upholding different deities as primary, there are clear philosophical differences in these three traditions. For example, Vaishnavism tends to emphasize the householder's life as the spiritual ideal and focuses on *videha-mukti*, or liberation after death, while Shaivism tends to emphasize the monastic or renunciate way of living as the ideal and focuses on seeking *jivan-mukti*, or liberation during life. But for all three, the primary textual repository for the legends, symbols, songs and ideas that give the tradition substance, form and beauty are the *Purānas*.

The Purānas

The word *Purāna* appears in the Vedas, though it's clear that the major and secondary Purānas commonly recognized today were compiled since the Vedic era. According to legend there was originally one *Purāna*, and it was compiled by Vyāsa, the same person who compiled the *Vedas* and narrates the *Mahābhārata*. The name *Vyāsa* means *compiler*, and in the yogic tradition there has actually been a reverse emphasis on authorship, with importance being placed on the scriptural authority of the text, specifically its relationship to other established texts, especially the *Vedas*, rather than on who wrote it.

Purāna essentially means *ancient*, and these texts are encyclopedic assimilations of Vedic and non-Vedic lore. They reflect the integration of the Vedic culture with local cultures as it spread throughout India over the course of centuries. There are eighteen *Mahāpurānas* (primary) and eighteen *Upapurānas* (secondary), and together they comprise over 400,000 verses. They are compilations of ancient wisdom and information that have been gathered, adapted, added to, reorganized, and rearranged.

They include everything from lists of dynastic successions to extensive mantras honoring particular deities, from recipes for cosmetics and astrological data to profound philosophical and metaphysical teachings, from specific information on grammar, minerals and pilgrimage sites to folk tales and love stories. There are several key stories that appear in many *Purānas*, sometimes with contextual differences that bring either Vishnu, Śiva, or Devī to the fore and emphasize their centrality. Many modern Hindu festivals, both local and national, are based on stories found in the *Purānas*, and a great deal of Indian art and music has been inspired by these beautiful and expansive texts.

The *Devī Bhagavata Purāṇa* is the main *Purāṇa* dedicated to the Divine Mother, and a central text of Shaktism. It is eighteen-thousand verses (more or less) and contains many stories in which Devī comes to the rescue of the devas by defeating a powerful demon. It also holds the 1,008 names of Devī, and a short section called the *Devī Gītā*, which is styled after the *Bhagavad Gītā* but features Devī as the teacher and the devas as her students.

Devīmāhātmya

But centuries before the *Devī Bhagavata Purāṇa* was compiled; another text central to Shaktism emerged and was popularized throughout India. The *Devīmāhātmya* is a section of the *Mārkandeya Purāṇa* in which the sage Mārkandeya shares three specific legends contained within a single story arc. The *Devīmāhātmya* articulates a profound philosophy that weaves together Vedantic non-duality and *bhakti* (devotion) to the Divine Mother. Four widely popular hymns with universal themes that contain deep wisdom and devotion come from this text: the *Brahmāstuti*, the *Śakrādistuti*, the *Aparājitāstuti*, and the *Nārāyaṇistuti*.

The *Devīmāhātmya* begins as Mārkandeya introduces the virtuous king Suratha, who has retired to a forest hermitage after losing his kingdom. Suratha soon meets the merchant Samādhi, who was rich and happy until his greedy family stole his wealth and cast him out. Both of them came to the forest retreat seeking peace, but find that in the quiet surroundings, they are faced with their attachment and pain of loss. Together they approach the sage Medhas, whose name signifies *insight*, and ask to be freed from the delusion that grips them. The sage replies that they have been "hurled into the whirlpool of attachment, the pit of delusion, by the power of Mahāmāya, who produces the continuing cycle of this transitory world." (All translations of the

Devīmāhātmya by Devādatta Kāli from the excellent book *In Praise of the Goddess.*)

The word *māyā* has entered our modern vocabulary, and it is often used in a pejorative sense. We think of it as a state to be escaped through practice leading to greater wisdom. But here Medhas refers to Mahāmāyā as the Divine Mother:

> *"She, the blessed goddess Mahāmāyā, seizes the minds of even the wise and draws them into delusion. She creates all this universe, moving and unmoving, and it is she who graciously bestows liberation on humanity. She is the supreme knowledge and the eternal cause of liberation, even as she is the cause of bondage to this transitory existence. She is the sovereign of all lords."*
>
> *(Devīmāhātmya 1.55-58)*

The king is confused by this and asks for clarification, and in reply Medhas tells the three stories about Devī.

In **Medhas' first story,** Brahmā has just been born out of Vishnu's naval while Vishnu sleeps on the eternal ocean. Suddenly, two fearsome asuras are born from Vishnu's earwax and come to devour Brahmā. Brahmā calls out for help to Yoganidrā, the Divine Mother, who is sleep. His beautiful prayer is the Brahmāstuti, which reveals Devī as the "nectar of immortality...the transcendent being...inseparable and inexpressible...the eternal source of all becoming...the supreme mother of the gods...the creative force at the world's birth and its sustenance for as long as it endures...the great knowledge and the great illusion, the great intelligence, the great memory, and the great delusion, the great goddess and the great demoness..."

Roused by the prayer, Devī awakens Vishnu, who battles with the demons for a century until they become prideful and make a mortal mistake. This ancient Vaishnava story has been changed to emphasize the role of Devī as Yoganidra:

> "Do not be astonished. This same Mahāmāyā is Yoganidrā, the meditative sleep of Vishnu, the lord of the world."
>
> (Devīmāhātmya 1.54)

Human life inherently involves limitation. Our eternal and infinite souls have consented to live in a world where we feel alone and separate, where the future is unknown, and where the primary stimulus for growth is pain. It's easy to feel resentful toward the state of limitation and see it as wrong or evil. But the *Devīmāhātmya* reminds us that limitation itself is the Divine Mother. Our limited consciousness is not a mistake, not our fault or a cause for shame or mockery. She lulls us into the sleep of egoistic delusion, in which we dream that we are small and finite. She conceals Her infinitude and grants us the experience of longing for Her, which draws Her progressively closer to us, and eventually joins us to Her in the embrace of yoga. This re-union is the hidden purpose of creation, and the goal toward which evolution climbs.

Medhas' second story recounts Durgā's victory over the dreaded Mahishasura. The demon Mahisha and his army have conquered Indra and the devas and cast them out of heaven. They come to Brahmā, Vishnu and Śiva asking for help, and a divine light radiates from the foreheads of the three great beings. This light is joined by light from all the other devas, which combines to create the fierce goddess Durgā, riding on a lion. Each of the devas gives her a weapon, and she single-handedly defeats the entire demon army and the buffalo-headed Mahishasura. After endlessly shape-shifting to escape Her, Durgā finally pins him down and pierces him with a spear, and his true form emerges from the mouth of the buffalo. Durgā Devī decapitates him with a single stroke.

In Durgā temples throughout India there are statues and paintings of Durgā on her lion standing on Mahisha's neck and piercing his side with a spear. And images of a goddess on a lion and a buffalo demon also appear on pre-Vedic artifacts from the Indus Valley in the modern Punjab. While the first story depicts Devī's tamasic aspect, the second shows her as *rajas*, the fire of swift action that conquers evil. Here Devī intervenes in the world to support the restoration of order and righteousness. Even as she enters the world of form and the field of battle where the asuras and devas struggle for supremacy, she remains calm, serene. She maintains her transcendent poise as she effortlessly defeats hordes of asuras. The countless arrows of Mahishasura's general Chiksura affect her as much as rain showers affect the primordial Mount Meru. His massive sword strikes her arm and shatters.

Devī is the protector, the mother lion who will face any foe to save her beloved children. When we are afraid, overwhelmed, despairing, when we have been cast from our homes and all seems lost, we can call out to Durgā Devī, cry for her protection from the depths of our hearts. And every call is heard, every cry receives Her loving reply. At the end of the second story, Indra and the gods sing Devī's praises in the Śakrādistuti and offer gratitude for her unconditional compassion. She slays the wicked who "may have committed enough evil to keep them long in torment" and redeems them so that they "may attain the higher worlds." No soul is beyond redemption, no evil act severs the link between Mother and child.

In the **third story**, Devī appears in her sattwic form as a beautiful woman. Again, two asuras, Śumbha, representing ego, and Niśumbha, attachment, have vanquished the devas and taken control of the three worlds: heaven, earth, and the underworld. The devas remember Devī's promise to respond to every sincere call, and so they call out to her in a profound prayer called the *Aparājitāstuti*. The prayer powerfully affirms that Devī abides within all beings as consciousness, intelligence, sleep, hunger, shadow, power, thirst, forgiveness, order, modesty, peace…and finally, even as error. When we experience ourselves as alone or unseen, it is only because she has veiled her presence within us.

In response to the prayer of the devas, Devī emerges from the body of Parvatī, who is traditionally the wife of Śiva, but in this story she is in no way subservient to anyone. When Śumbha and Niśumbha's spies Chanda and Munda see the resplendent form of Devī, they rush back to tell the demon kings about her. They are immediately gripped with desire and a need to possess her. Her reply to their advances is that only one who has defeated her in battle can marry her. Again, Devī defeats layers of armies and generals, including Raktabīja, who replicates himself anew every time a drop of his blood touches the Earth. Devī manifests the fearsome Kālī to catch each bead of blood in midair. "And within her mouth those great asuras who sprang into being from the flow, those she now devoured, even while drinking Raktabīja's blood."

Śumbha is the naked ego, captivated by the Divine One and her awesome power, but only wanting that power for himself. His brother Niśumbha is attachment, and walks always in front, grasping and clutching that which the ego desires. These brothers are powerful and confident, cunning and elusive, and they approach Devī and accuse her of cheating by creating the various forms that fought on her behalf. In reply, she draws the emanations back into herself and utters what is considered a *mahāvākya*, or great dictum: "I am alone here in the world. Who else is there besides me?"

In the end, Devī defeats the force of ego represented by Śumbha. "When the evil one was slain, all the universe became calm, regaining its natural order, and the sky cleared." She has liberated the soul, and it radiates light and truth without the interference of ego, which distorts perception and clouds vision. When we embark on a spiritual path, often the initial motivation is a combination of an emergent soul longing for freedom and the ego's desire for spiritual power. Lusting for self-enhancement, the ego can grow stronger through the cultivation of spiritual wisdom and authority. But ultimately it must face Devī, who is immune to the ego's false power.

Sri Aurobindo and the Divine Mother

Sri Aurobindo reminds us that Devī is both the transcendent One to whom we reach to escape the suffering round of life and death, and the Mother who nurtures evolution and draws all beings toward wholeness. His teachings proclaim that the world is not a mistake from which we must escape. The world is purposeful, and evolution moves ceaselessly toward fulfillment of the Divine Plan. To participate in fulfilling this plan, Sri Aurobindo encourages us to surrender our entire selves at the feet of the Divine Mother, and to ask Her to take us up as an instrument for Her great work. He sees the Mother as an evolutionary force that flows through the forces of nature to bring about greater enlightenment for all beings:

> *"If you want to be a true doer of divine works, your first aim must be to be totally free from all desire and self-regarding ego. All your life must be an offering and a sacrifice to the Supreme; your only object in action shall be to serve, to receive, to fulfill, to become a manifesting instrument of the Divine Shakti in her works. You must grow in the divine consciousness till there is no difference between your will and hers, no motive except her*

impulsion in you, no action that is not her conscious action in you and through you."

(from The Mother, by Sri Aurobindo)

We often think of surrender as a struggle, an effort that we make to give up something important. But in this case, what we are giving up is the ego's false importance, and what we gain instead is the freedom of the soul to act in accordance with its true nature. When we stand separate in our individuality, enforcing our small will upon the world, then we live in a constant state of struggle and suffering. But when we surrender this small will and join with the Mother's vast and perfect Will, we receive joy and peace beyond measure.

> *"A time will come when you will feel more and more that you are the instrument and not the worker. For first by the force of your devotion your contact with the Divine Mother will become so intimate that at all times you will have only to concentrate and to put everything into her hands to have her present guidance, her direct command or impulse, the sure indication of the thing to be done and the way to do it and the result. And afterwards you will realise that the divine Shakti not only inspires and guides, but initiates and carries out your works; all your movements are originated by her, all your powers are hers; mind, life and body are conscious and joyful instruments of her action, means for her play, moulds for her manifestation in the physical universe. There can be no more happy condition than this union and dependence; for this step carries you back beyond the borderline from the life of stress and suffering in the ignorance into the truth of your spiritual being, into its deep peace and its intense Ananda."*

(from The Mother, by Sri Aurobindo)

In modern yoga, this unequivocal surrender has been supplanted by a doctrine of ego empowerment. We are encouraged to feel powerful, in control, to work hard and gain strength, flexibility, stamina. The ancient teachings of yoga do of course encourage strength and courage, but always and only in service to our deepening of the union of spirit and matter, identification with our soul, and devotion to the Supreme One. Modern western yoga is rife with false teachings that have cloaked themselves in yogic dress, and instead of encouraging the surrender of the ego's desires at the feet of the Divine, actually encourage building the ego's fortress and glittering city of glamor. We must be scrupulous in our *viveka* (discernment), as these teachings have a subtle way of weaving themselves into a scenery that we take for granted.

In his condensed articulation of the heart of Shaktism, a small booklet called *The Mother*, Sri Aurobindo describes four powers of the Divine Mother, "four of her outstanding Personalities, portions, and embodiments of her divinity." These four are reflected in the Mother's Symbol as the four central petals around an inner circle. The inner circle represents Aditi, "the one original transcendent Shakti" who also "enters into the worlds she has made; her presence fills and supports them with the divine spirit...without which they could not exist." The four petals represent Maheshwari, Mahākali, Mahālakshmī, and Mahāsaraswatī.

Maheshwarī is "the mighty and wise One who opens us to...the cosmic vastness, to the grandeur of the Supreme Light...Tranquil is she and wonderful, great and calm forever...[S]he is above all, bound by nothing, attached to nothing in the universe. Yet has she more than any other the heart of the universal Mother. For her compassion is endless and inexhaustible."

Mahākali is "of another nature…not wisdom but force and strength are her peculiar power. There is in her an overwhelming intensity, a mighty passion of force to achieve, a divine violence rushing to shatter every limit and obstacle. Terrible is her face to the Asura, dangerous and ruthless her mood against the haters of the Divine… [S]he smites awake at once with sharp pain, if need be, the untimely slumberer and the loiterer."

Mahālakshmī is "the miracle of eternal beauty, an unseizable secret of divine harmonies…and there is no aspect of the Divine Shakti more attractive to the heart of embodied things. For she throws the spell of intoxicating sweetness of the Divine: to be close to her is a profound happiness, and to feel her within the heart is to make existence a rapture and a marvel."

Mahāsaraswatī is "the Mother's Power of Work and her spirit of perfection and order. This Power is the strong, the tireless, the careful and efficient builder, organizer, administrator, technician, artisan and crafter of the worlds…[L]eaning over us she notes and touches every little detail, finds out every minute defect, gap, twist or incompleteness…Nothing is too small or apparently trivial for her attention…Therefore of all the Mother's powers she is the most long suffering with [us] and [our] thousand imperfections. Kind, smiling, close and helpful, not easily turned away or discouraged, insistent even after repeated failure, her hand sustains our every step on condition that we are single in our will and straightforward and sincere, for…her revealing irony is merciless to drama and histrionics and self-deceit and pretense."

These four powers are present throughout the universe, in the cosmos and in our lives. They await our prayers, our outreach. Through them we can connect to the primordial Devī and invite Her grace into our hearts and our days. And if we are willing to surrender the immediate and impulsive desires of our egoic nature, we can become Her instruments in the great and difficult work of cosmic evolution. And this is the ultimate fulfillment and satisfaction toward which all desire yearns.

Reverence, Compassion, and Care

Along with surrender, the Divine Mother encourages reverence for all that is. She pervades all of existence, inhabiting everything, and asks us to look for her within all beings with reverence and honoring. Reverence is a gift that we offer to ourselves. It is deeply nourishing, calming, and transformative. It's like a balm for the soul that longs to express the truth of its relationship with all that is.

We can revere and honor the One Transcendent Being that exists beyond creation, or the Universal Divine whose body is the manifest universe, or the indwelling Divine that resides within every individual. We can bow to a mountain, a statue, a painting, or a person. It's not the form that matters, it's the inner experience. Bowing is like medicine, and it's the perfect remedy for a society that is sick with the delusion of ego aggrandizement.

Bowing also reinforces the truth that, as Sri Aurobindo reminds us, we should not try to "understand and judge the Divine Mother by [the] little earthly mind that loves to subject even the things that are beyond it to its own norms and standards, its narrow reasoning and erring impressions, its bottomless aggressive ignorance and its petty self-confident knowledge." Reverence empowers humility, without which we cannot approach Truth in any form.

Along with reverence comes compassion and care. When we see the Divine Mother within all of creation, then we cannot help caring for the Earth, for all creatures great and small, and for each other. If we are all parts of the Mother's body, if we are all Her children, then no one is outside of our human family – no one is undeserving of our love and care. Many of us feel primarily responsible for our own family, and honor our own human mother because she gave us the gift of life. Without in any way diminishing these feelings, the Divine Mother calls us to experience ourselves as Her child, and to widen our sense of family to include all of humanity and all of creation.

And so, true yoga requires a subservience of our own self-centered desires, bowing to and serving all beings. There's nothing linear about this, as we each have our own unique dhārma to fulfill on behalf of all, but it does mean that finding our *dhārma* will always include taking care of others and loosening the hold of our self-fixation. And that means facing ourselves and the fears that fuel egoism. But we don't do this alone. The Mother of the Universe, the Great Cosmic Mother Whose sight is perfect, Who knows all and bears all, is right there with us. She feels our every pain and fear, She holds us through every trial, and She never turns away for even a breath.

> *"Remembered in distress, you remove fear from every creature. Remembered by the untroubled, you confer even greater serenity of mind. Dispeller of poverty, suffering and fear, who, other than you, is ever intent on benevolence toward all?"*
>
> (Devīmāhātmya 4.17)

Chapter - 9

Thirumanthiram and Tantrāloka – Gifts of Śiva

It's dark, before dawn, and the streets of Tiruvannamalai are quiet, but not silent. Dogs bark, cows chew through piles of garbage, and mantra music drifts out of loudspeakers from various shrines and temples. I've been walking for an hour, and I still feel fresh, alive. I turn to the right, and across the street I see the top of the holy Arunāchala Hill in the distance. My heart rejoices at the sight.

Arunāchala is the embodiment of Śiva, the holy outcaste, the compassionate one who takes upon himself all the refuse that no one else wants. Arunāchala is his radiant form, shining upon the world as a mountain that dominates the landscape for miles around. The Girivalam Path, the circumambulation route around the base of Arunāchala that I've been walking, is over eight miles long. It has been a pilgrimage path since before humans could write. For me, it's a way of greeting Arunāchala, of honoring and revering this sacred mountain that lives within my heart.

I stop and sit by the side of the road. On the sidewalk next to me is a man wearing the orange robes of renunciation, with dreadlocks, a salt and pepper beard, and a collection of rudraksha malas strung around his neck. He holds a book and chants verses in Tamil, songs of adoration to Śiva and Arunāchala. I absorb the vibration of his words, I take in the beauty of the mountain through my eyes and through my heart, and I offer myself, my life, my thoughts, my sense of purpose, to the Divine One that lives within all hearts. "Take me, show me, guide me," I pray, and I feel the answer flow through my breath and body, wrapping all that I am in the Divine embrace.

History

Śiva's historical roots are unclear. Perhaps the Vedic Rudra, the howling storm with his wild band of Maruts, merged with the pre-Vedic Bhairava, the "lord of the hunt." Some scholars believe that 10,000+ year old carvings found in caves in Madhya Pradesh depict Śiva dancing, carrying his trident, and his bull Nandi. The adjective śiva is applied to many different devas in the Rig Veda, and has the sense of auspiciousness, kindness, graciousness, and benevolence. But it is not used as the name of a specific divine being until the Śvetashvatara Upanishad, which was probably written in the few centuries before the advent of the Common Era.

What is clear is that throughout the first millennium CE, Śaivism as a spiritual framework expanded throughout India, and most of India's various traditions that fall under the modern category of *Hinduism* acknowledge Śiva as a deva of great importance. The *Trimurti*, or triple being, is fundamental to most Hindu traditions; it includes Brahmā the creator, Vishnu the preserver, and Śiva the destroyer. In Vaishnava traditions, Vishnu is the embodiment of the Divine Singularity, the Highest Soul, and Śiva is His ardent devotee. In Śaiva traditions, Śiva is the Ultimate, the unreachable yet pervasive Supreme that created the others.

The Imminent, Transcendent One

Śiva reconciles all opposites. He transcends and stands apart from creation, alone and pure, and simultaneously he permeates the universe; every molecule of creation emanates from Him and is infused by His essence. He IS the universe, the truth, the falsehood, the joy, the agony, the love, the enmity. Nothing escapes Him. Nothing is not Himself.

Śiva is the lone wanderer, the ascetic meditating in the dense forest and on the mountaintop, in the cremation grounds and in the earthy cave. He is *alinga*: formless and without cause. He is unreachable, aloof. Wild dreaded *jata* (dreadlocks) tangle around the crescent moon that rests on His head. Smeared with ash, cobras draping His shoulders and a skull for a begging bowl, He is Bhairava. He is Natarāja, and He dances the *tandava*: the creation, sustenance and dissolution of all forms, the dance of birth and death that haunts our days. He is Rudra, the howler, the hurricane, and Tryambakam, the three-eyed one who pervades the universe like a scent, who offers, but also often withholds, the gift of release.

Śiva is inseparable from Śakti. He is eternally joined with Satī, Pārvatī, Maheśvarī. Without Her power and force, without His beloved, He is nothing, the universe is nothing, not even the endless void. His heart is joined with Hers, and when She destroys Herself to save his honor, He is lost in rage, invoking Vīrabhadra to avenge Her death. Heartbroken and desolate, He recommits to his solitary tapas, but Uma, daughter of the ancient Himalayas, re-incarnation of Sati, avatar of Śakti, heals Him, reminds Him what it is to be loved. When He drank the Halāhala poison that threatened to destroy all life, She clamped His throat shut to save Him, and thus saved the universe, which floats in His stomach. Śakti and Śiva are One, Ardhanārīśvara, complete in their union they give birth to all worlds. She is His body and breath, and He is Her essence, Her timeless self.

Śiva is the Jyotirlinga, the endless pillar of pure light, too tall for Brahmā to climb, too deep for Vishnu to dig. He is the holy mountain *Arunāchala*, radiating the fire of purification and release, calling pilgrims and sadhus from around the world. He is the self-referential ego, the sense that "I am all that matters," that "What happens to me is more important than your pain, your trouble, your fear." He is the need to control, the delusion of self-isolation, the *ahankara: I maker*. He is the *spanda*, the subtle vibration that underlies everything. He is everything: *sarvāya*.

Thirumanthiram: God Is Love

Throughout most of the first millennium, Śaiva spirituality was dualistic, emphasized worship of Śiva without Śakti, focused on ritual as the primary *upāya*, or means to liberation, and aligned with the norms of Vedic society as dictated by *brāhmin* priests. This tradition was known as Śaiva Siddhānta. But even within the foundations of this tradition, tantric mysticism was present. Tirumular's *Thirumanthiram*, or "Holy Incantation," which was likely written in the first few centuries CE, is a root text of Śaiva Siddhānta, and expresses reverence for its common traditions. But it is clearly a *tantrik* text, meaning that it reveals a practical mysticism that shares the essential features of **tantrik** traditions listed in the next section below.

Tirumular was one of the sixty-three Tamil *Nayanars*, or *hounds of Śiva*, the main proponents of Śiva bhakti in Tamil Nadu during the first millennium CE. These poet/singer saints gave themselves to devotion and expounded a doctrine of loving surrender to Śiva as a path to liberation. They found divine bliss, and sought to share it with the world: "May this world share the bliss that I have had" (*Thirumanthiram*). The legend goes that a yogi named Sundarar was living on Mount Kailas in the Himalayas. On a journey south, he noticed a herd of cows gathered around the body of their cowherd, Mulan, and crying miserably. Out of compassion for the cows, Sundarar left his own body and entered that of Mulan, who immediately came to life. Sundarar, in the body of Mulan, took the cows home and then came back for his own body, which had disappeared, having been stolen by Śiva himself. The yogi/cowherd sat beneath a peepul tree and entered a deep meditative state. Eventually he came to be known by the local people as Tirumular (holy Mulan), and they would sit and wait for him to periodically emerge from Samādhi and utter a few verses, which they recorded. In all they took down three-thousand verses, which form the *Thirumanthiram*.

Thirumanthiram is the earliest known of the Tamil *tantrik* texts. It was composed in poetic meter and covers a wide range of topics, including metaphysics, mantras and yantras, references to Patañjali's 8-limbed yoga, and the means to attain *kaya siddhi*, or a perfected and immortal body. But its central message is *Anbe Śivam*: Love is Śiva. Śiva is source and inner being of everything – He did not create the universe as something apart from Himself; He became the universe, or more appropriately, He is constantly becoming the universe. And Love is Śiva, the inner self of all.

> *The ignorant rant that Love and Śiva are two,*
> *They know not that Love alone is Śiva*
> *When we learn that Love and Śiva are the same*
> *Love as Śiva, they ever remain.*
>
> – *Thirumanthiram 270*

> *Worship the Lord with heart melted in love;*
> *Seek the Lord with love,*
> *When we direct our love to God*
> *He too approaches us with love.*
>
> - *Thirumanthiram 275*

Yama, Niyama, and Asana numberless
Prānāyāma and Pratyahara wholesome and pure
Triumphant Dhāranā, Dhyāna, and Samādhi
These eight are the steely limbs of Yoga.
- Thirumanthiram 552

This is the way to chant: Śivaya Nama, Śivaya Nama
If you chant this way, birth will come no more
With Lord's Grace, you shall behold the Eternal Dance
And copper jiva becomes gold Śiva.
- Thirumanthiram 906

Having learned all there is to learn
And practiced all the possible Yogas
Then they pursue the graded path of jñana
And so pass into the world of formless sound
There, rid of all impurities, they envision the supreme, the self-created: They are the true Śaiva Siddhantas.
- Thirumanthiram 1421

Offer the flower of 'you' at the feet of 'He';
Then no more will you speak of 'you' and 'He'.
Thirumanthiram 1607

Over the centuries, Śaiva Siddhānta became concentrated mostly in South India, and integrated Śankara's Advaita Vedānta (non-dual) philosophy. Today Śaiva Siddhanta essentially exists only in Tamil Nadu (India's southernmost state), and its philosophy remains non-dualistic. In India, spirituality is rooted in the earth and in sacred space. There are several temples and sacred sites throughout Tamil Nadu connected to Śiva, including Ramanathaswamy Temple in Ramesvaram, where Rām prayed to Śiva for redemption after killing the demon king Rāvana. One of the main lingams inside the temple sanctum is said to have been built out of sand by Ram's wife Sītā herself. The *Cidambarām Nataraja Temple* honors Śiva's dance and its qualities of both creation/destruction and sensuality, and is the origin of the ubiquitous *Nataraja* statue.

Arunāchala and Subjective Spiritual Experience

Arunāchala is the Sanskrit name of a hill in Tiruvannamalai that has been honored since time immemorial as the physical body of Śiva. The sacred mountain radiates grace, and millions of pilgrims come each year from around the world seeking blessings and transformation. Sri Ramana Mahārshi is the most famous of many saints who have been drawn to *Arunāchala,* or *Annamalai* in Tamil (the local language), and given themselves to the mountain. He shared the mountain's energy and message with the world through his teachings. But many others came before him, like Guhai Namaśivāya, who meditated in a cave on the mountainside until his soul left his body and split the giant rock above him. And others have come since, like Swami Nārāyana, who recently lived for eighteen years right beside the summit under a canvas tarp, rarely spoke or walked, and survived almost entirely on milk brought to the summit by devotees. Today saints and seekers continue to come to *Arunāchala,* drawn by Śiva's presence. They join themselves to the sacred vibration that radiates from the mountain and participate in its radiance.

> *Arunāchala is truly the holy place. Of all holy places it is the most sacred! Know that it is the heart of the world. It is truly Śiva himself! It is his heart-abode, a secret kshetra. In that place the Lord ever abides as the hill of light named Arunāchala.*
> – Sri Rāmana Mahārshi

Arunāchala Śiva invites us into relationship; it calls out to be experienced. When we see it in a photo, or walk the eight-mile pilgrimage route around it, when we sit in its caves or stand on its summit, we have the opportunity to experience the heart of Arunāchala Śiva. But too frequently, we deny our own spiritual experiences. Or perhaps more often, our beliefs about what's possible are so strong and rigid that they don't even allow us to accept that we're having a spiritual experience at all. It's like sitting outside in the sun and not feeling the warmth because the forecast called for cold. Or perhaps the person next to us says "You're crazy, it's not warm! It's cold." Who do we trust? Our own experience of warmth? Or the others who deny it?

The scientific method has served us profoundly in penetrating the manipulation of spiritual truth by elites. But it has also stripped us of our own subjectivity. It has subjugated our own freedom of experience to "experts" and machines. If we happen to have an experience that contradicts what's commonly accepted as possible or verifiable, we risk being mocked and discredited. This need not be so. We can be scientifically scrupulous in our exploration of our own inner experiences, if we remain open and flexible enough for those experiences to manifest and touch our awareness.

The good news is that no belief system or social pressure can actually revoke, or even diminish spiritual experience. Experiences persist, sometimes below the surface of what our conscious awareness will allow, sometimes poking through and challenging the status quo of our own belief systems. They persist because, as the saying goes, Truth will out. What is real cannot stay hidden beneath the veil of falsehood forever. So when Arunāchala Śiva, or any other spiritually alive entity, calls to you, the message is always received.

The original dualistic Śaiva Siddhānta philosophies considered the Divine, the creation, and the individual as distinctly and eternally separate. The world of birth, life and death was considered to be like a prison from which only God's grace could offer liberation. Liberation came in the form of a guru, who would offer initiation and mystically empowered mantras that would lead toward freedom, but not union with the Divine, who is forever separate from all individual souls. This dualistic Śaiva Siddhānta tradition was one of the first emergences of what we now call *tantra*.

Tantra: Practical Mysticism

The word *tantra* is possibly even more misunderstood in the west than the word *Yoga*. In the early twentieth century, an American named Pierre Bernard learned some basic *tantrik* principles from an Indian immigrant, and founded the first *tantrik* sex cult. Interestingly, *tantrik* sex rituals are mentioned in one text out of hundreds of ancient *tantrik* texts, and even these rituals are not aimed at maximizing pleasure. What has come to be known as neo-tantra today is not really neo-anything, but an invention of the modern west that ties itself to tantra for validation, and that has flourished in an ecosystem where sexuality and feminine principles have been suppressed and repressed.

The word *tantra* has the basic sense of *doctrine* or *book*, and the *tantrik* tradition arose in India during the sixth century CE, coalescing around specific texts that were considered divine revelations of a new spirituality that was more practically appropriate for the time at hand. Just like the Vedas and *Upanishads* before them, the *Tantras* were considered a gift of the Divine One, in this case to help humanity cope with the suffering that arises from the naturally declining morality of the *kali yuga*. Over the centuries, thousands of *tantras*, also sometimes called āgamas, or *that which was passed down*, have been written, and their general focus has been on specific practices and rituals that prepare one for liberation, or *moksha*.

Defining tantra broadly as a movement is difficult, and several scholars have developed lists of the key features common to most tantrik traditions, which minimally includes Śaiva Tantra, *Buddhist Tantra*, and *Vaishnava Tantra*. Christopher Wallis, in his excellent book *Tantra Illuminated*, compiled a list that combines other lists, and below are a few highlights:

- Alternative path, new revelation, more rapid path
- Centrality of ritual, especially the evocation and worship of deities
- Visualization and self-identification with deities
- Use of *mantras*, *yantras*, *mandalas*, yoga, and linguistic mysticism
- Necessity of initiation and importance of esotericism/secrecy
- Spiritual physiology (i.e. subtle body and *chakras*) and *kundalini*
- Importance of the teacher (guru, ācārya)
- Lay/householder practitioners
- Importance of śakti (power, energy, goddess) and valuing the status and role of women
- Revaluation of the body and "negative" mental states

This list comprises both dual and non-dual *tantrik* traditions, although the last two items apply particularly to non-dual and *left-hand path* streams. More on the *left-hand path* in a bit.

So essentially *tantra* was the secret, practical mysticism that grew out of and responded to the major Indian religious movements. Today many western teachers will connect the word tantra to the metaphor of weaving, but Wallis asserts that this is just a homonym, and is never actually used in any tantrik text, though it does fit with the spirit of the movement as a whole. Although even defining a "movement as a whole" is a tricky business. "In medieval India, those people who received *tantrik* initiation usually received it from a single guru in a specific lineage and performed the daily practice given by that guru on the basis of a single tantra. So for each individual practitioner, Tantra as a spiritual movement was not something highly complex." *Tantrikas* were concerned with their own *guru*/**śishya**, or teacher/disciple relationship, their own practice and liberation.

Guru: A Guide on the Path

In eight-hundred CE, it wasn't possible to skip down to the local bookstore and purchase a *tantrik* text, and then go home and get started on your liberation. A guru was an unequivocal necessity in *tantra*. During the initial flourishing of *tantra*, when the Śaiva Siddhānta tradition was expanding throughout India, there was a distinction between regular people going about their lives, fulfilling their social roles and performing their inherited socio-religious rituals, and *tantrikas*, who were accepted by a *guru* and initiated into the secret tradition. Generally, before seeking out a *guru*, a person would have an experience of śaktipāta, or a descent of divine energy that awakens the inner being. This śaktipāta experience could be intense, immediate, and violent, or it could evolve more gradually over time, but it essentially was an inner process of awakening that signaled the beginning of a spiritual quest, not its end.

After a śaktipāta experience, one would seek out, or perhaps synchronistically encounter, a *guru*. The guru would take on the task of supporting the integration of that experience and expanding on it, peeling away layers of delusion to reveal greater and greater degrees of truth. Because of the ego's nature, it was understood that facing oneself is not possible without a *guru's* direction, support and care. There were rare cases in which the *guru* role was fulfilled by an inner relationship with the Divine, but this Divine Being was experienced as separate from the ego-self throughout the process of initiation, progressive integration, and liberation.

This is an area where things in the west have gotten very mixed up. We long for truth, we aspire to know ourselves and uncover our true nature. And we are surrounded by countless books, movies, podcasts, facebook posts, and every other kind of information package. Voices assail us to buy, subscribe, join and gain what we are looking for. Simultaneously, we hear endless stories of gurus who have manipulated their position, taken advantage of their power, and victimized their community. This combination of forces compels us to seek to control our spiritual path, so we don't fall into the wrong hands. But the problem is that any real spiritual path will absolutely require a release of control. Control and liberation are diametrically opposed.

The reality is that we are not afraid of being deceived by a false guru. We are afraid of our own smallness. We are afraid that there is no Divine Being guiding our path, and that if we fall in a hole or off a cliff, it's because we failed. This is not the message of Śiva. Śiva leads us down dark passageways, into the depth of the moonless night, to the cremation grounds where we face our own mortality. Śiva's grace is the release of the impulse to control, and this process is never straightforward or predictable. Opening to Śiva means stepping out into the unknown and facing our fears, taking risks in trusting our own discernment.

When we want something for ourselves, when the ego has manipulated our spiritual longing into a self-aggrandizing desire, we are vulnerable to manipulation by others. When we grasp for something that will make us feel bigger, better, smarter, stronger, then whoever offers us that golden chalice assumes a false power over us. But when we surrender our self, when we make an offering of the ego and its desires, then the inner light of discernment will guide us by a path that we know not. We will be carried, and even when we are engulfed by the deepest impenetrable darkness, we will move inexorably forward.

The true *guru* will appear, the one whose love is pure and without need, the one whose heart is whole and has nothing to gain or lose.

Kashmir Śaiva Tantra

Over the centuries, hundreds, if not thousands of streams of *tantra* evolved. In some way, although they relied on shared texts that maintained some philosophical integrity, each individual *guru* led each individual *sadhāka* (aspirant) on their own unique path. Over time, philosophical streams emerged, converged, and defined themselves, and broader communities formed around a set of teachings, practices and cosmologies. Some of these communities tended to align with the Vedic orthodoxy and affirm the social norms of the day. Others deviated slightly from conventional norms, and still others directly spurned the status quo.

These distinctions came to be known as the "right-hand path" and the "left-hand path." Right-hand communities tended to be dualistic and conformist, with *gurus* who were more like officiants. They didn't need to be "awakened" themselves, as long as they were educated about the ritualistic structures that they needed to teach. Left-hand communities moved in the direction of non-dualism, worship of the feminine, inclusion of women, transgression of social norms, and charismatic gurus who had directly experienced the non-dual nature of reality and could transmit their experiences to their students directly. The most extreme left-hand communities performed rituals that directly transgressed social norms, and even included practices that most people would consider disgusting. One purpose of these practices was to break down the idea that Śiva only lives as things that we consider clean or palatable, and open consciousness to the indwelling divinity in everything. And like all *tantrik* practices, they were also meant to strip the individual of the self-referential stories that come to define us and inhibit the experience of our own divinity.

The Śaiva Tantra traditions, especially the "left-hand path," were influenced by early Śiva-worshipping groups like the *Paśupatis*, who took the *mahāvrata*, or "Great Vow." These yogis imitated Bhairava, a fierce and fearsome form of Śiva, by wandering naked, smeared with ash, and begged for food using a bowl made from a human skull. They meditated around funeral pyres in cremation grounds and often acted insane. Significantly, these ascetics were voluntarily assuming a lifestyle that was the common punishment for someone who committed the worst sin of all – murdering a *brāhmin* priest. They intentionally placed themselves completely outside of society to establish complete independence and freedom from a socially defined self.

In general, our self-concept is small. Our basic experience of self, made up of beliefs and stories that repetition weaves into a sturdy fabric, diminishes us. We think and behave as if we are only capable of loving so much, of giving so much, before we run out. We don't feel capable of fully giving ourselves to Love, to Life, to serving humanity or the Divine. We experience ourselves as finite and so we protect and hoard. But according to Śaiva Tantra traditions, we are not finite at all, and there is nothing we need to protect or hold onto. Our essential nature is Śiva, Whose freedom is limitless, and Whose very infinite nature is Love itself.

These right and left-hand traditions did agree on this: that ignorance veils our true divine nature, and this is the root of human suffering. They all also considered the *tantrik* texts to be divine revelations, given by Śiva out of compassion to point the way to liberation. The texts provide the framework for an initiation ceremony that someone who had received a śaktipāta would go through. A *guru* would look for signs of true śaktipāta before taking on a student, and then would conduct the ceremony, essentially standing in for Śiva, who is the real ceremonial officiant. During the ritual, all previous karma that would inhibit spiritual growth was burned up, opening the path to freedom.

Generally, the right-hand path traditions were more homogeneous, while the left-hand path traditions were less institutionalized and thus harder to summarize or define categorically. Over time the name *kaula*, or "from the family," arose to group left-hand-leaning *tantrik* traditions, which interestingly would not have called themselves *tantrik*. That's because the sense of the word *tantrik* has the feeling of ritualism, and while these traditions employed rituals in their seeking of liberation, they saw themselves as transcending the dogmatic application of set rituals and expanding, reworking, and recontextualizing rituals as needed for the case at hand.

In northwest India, in the area known as Kashmir, a particular branch of *Kaula Tantra* developed that has come to be known as *Kashmir Śaivism*. During the last century of the first millennium, the *tantrik* lineage became connected with the royal court. As a result, many highly educated people were initiated and introduced to the tradition. The writings that come from this time are powerful, sophisticated, and incisively clear, and they also had the benefit of royal benefactors who ensured that they were preserved and honored, even revered. These writings, some commentaries on original *tantrik* texts and others original *tantrik* treatises in their own right, were rooted in the ancient *tantrik* teachings, but introduced new elements that distinguished a coherent school.

Abhinava Gupta's Tantrasāra: Remembering Who We Are

One teacher from this period stands out as a luminary and grand synthesizer – his name is Abhinava Gupta. He wrote a great deal, and his most comprehensive and significant work is called *Tantrāloka*, which lays out a framework that integrates philosophy and practice and synthesizes several apparently contradictory schools of thought. Much of what we think of today as the philosophy of *Kashmir Śaivism* traces back to Abhinava Gupta's *Tantrāloka*. Because it is so comprehensive and intricate, and because of Abhinava Gupta's desire to share the healing truth as widely as possible, he also composed a condensed version of the *Tanrāloka* called *Tantrasāra* (the essence of *tantra*).

As everyone is not capable of delving deep into the long text of the Tantrāloka, this Tantrasāra is composed in simple language. Therefore, please listen to it. – Tantrasāra 1.2 (translation by H.N. Chakravarty)

A significant assertion of these texts is that liberation comes from recognizing and experiencing our true nature as Śiva; we don't need to become something different in order to be free; we don't need to improve ourselves; we just need to remember who we already are.

> *In this world, innate nature (svabhava) is the highest aim to be attained. This svabhava belonging to all entities is of the nature of light (prakaśa)...[and] that prakaśa is indeed only one, and that prakaśa alone is consciousness...The shining of that prakaśa is not dependent on anything outside of itself... there is only this single and autonomous prakaśa.*
> – *Tantrasāra, Introduction (translation by H.N. Chakravarty)*

> *The Self (ātmā) is prakaśa free from the limitations of thought constructs, and is the very nature of Śiva.*
> – *Tantrasāra, Chapter 1 Commentary (translation by H.N. Chakravarty)*

> *[Śiva] himself, as a result of his own freedom, binds himself here by means of actions whose nature are composed of imagined differentiations. Such is the power of the God's freedom that, even though he has become the finite self, he once more truly attains his own true form in all its purity.*
> – Tantrāloka 13.103-104 (translation by Paul Muller Ortega)

Another major assertion is that our limitless and pure essential being, which is Śiva, has freely taken on impurity, which is the root of our suffering. *Tantrik* practices offer us a means of purification, of clearing that which obscures our vision. This purification is not a task taken on by the ego in order to become cleaner, or to become more worthy of love. It is a submission of the ego to a process that strips its reinforced self-delusion and opens the way to an experience of the actual purity that is the Self's true nature. Thoughts that support the experience of separation and isolation are purified, and since these thoughts are understood to be deeply rooted in the body, the purification process includes physical purification, though not necessarily by external means. For purification to truly occur, the aspirant must surrender the personal will to a higher power, since the ego will never offer itself to be cleansed of falsehood, and will use powerful manipulations to remain concealed.

> *The lack of right knowledge (ajñana) is explained in the holy texts to be the cause of bondage. It is known as impurity (mala). At the rise of perfect knowledge it is uprooted in its entirety. Upon the emergence of Self-consciousness, at the time when all malas are destroyed, release (moksha) is attained."*
> – Tantrasāra, Introduction (translation by H.N. Chakravarty)

> *The very nature of consciousness is its freedom from thought constructs (vikalpa)...Listening to this nature of the Self*

> *repeatedly, thinking of it, and meditating on it continuously, help the vikalpa to become purified...With the purification of vikalpas, in the right manner, consciousness shines forth with all its glory.*
> – H.N. Chakravarty's footnote to Chapter 4 of his Tantrasāra translation

Abhinava Gupta also wrote a short meditation manual called the *Parātrīśika-laghuvritti*, which focuses on the Heart mantra *SAUH*. Paul Muller-Ortega's book *The Triadic Heart of Śiva* explores this text and the focus on the Heart in *Kashmir Śaiva Tantra* generally. Abhinava Gupta speaks of the Heart as the One Itself, the container of all creation, and the intermediary zone between the One and the many. The Heart is the ultimate reality, the transcendent, as well as our human faculty for perceiving the truth, for touching our own essence. It is beyond, *anuttara*, and also *madhya*, the center of our being. It is the embodied cosmos: every substance, every sensation, every emotion, every thought, every belief, every action and reaction – all happens within the Heart and all is an interaction of the Heart with Itself. It governs inspiration, intuition, direct knowing, receiving grace.

Always new, hidden, yet old and apparent to all, the Heart, the Ultimate shines alone with the brilliance of the Supreme. – Introductory verse of the Parātrīśika-laghuvritti (translation by Paul Muller-Ortega)

Just as the massive tree sleeps as potential within the banyan seed, so this world, both inanimate and animate, abides in the seed of the Heart. - Parātrīśika-laghuvritti, śloka 24b-25a (translation by Paul Muller-Ortega)

The centrality of the Heart defies the modern western tendency to intellectualize spirituality. We think we can find illumination through the mind, that we can think our way to enlightenment, or collect enough ideas and theories to wake ourselves up. But without the Heart, our spirituality is dry, brittle, lifeless. Attending to our Heart shifts us from thinking to feeling, from ideas to experiences, from theories to realities. The mind reaches for truth but can never grasp it. The Heart knows truth through resonance, because its nature is truth.

Modern Postural Yoga

As Christopher Wallis emphasizes in *Tantra Illuminated*, while we tend to think of modern postural yoga as arising from *Patañjali's Yoga Sūtras*, much more of the actual substance of the practice is rooted in *tantra*. For one thing, the main texts of *hatha yoga*, including the Śiva Samhitā, the *Gheranda Samhitā*, and the *Hatha Yoga Pradipika* (which is mostly a compilation of earlier works), are essentially *tantrik* texts. And the application of asanas, mudras and mantras to specific physiological and psychological conditions is clearly a *tantrik* approach.

Beyond this, most of the major streams of modern yoga can be traced back to a man named Tirumalai Krishnamacharya. He taught B.K.S. Iyengar, Pattabhi Jois, T.K.V. Desikachar, and Indra Devi, all of whom had a momentous impact on the development and spread of yoga in the west. Krishnamacharya studied yoga and *Sankhya* philosophy as a youth, and held advanced degrees in all six *darśanas*, or major philosophical schools of Hinduism. When he was just 16, he fell into a trance and was given a direct dictation of an ancient text called *Yoga Rahasya* by its original author Nathamuni. He had become a well-known yoga teacher before he traveled by foot to Tibet to study with the *tantrik* guru Yogeshwara Ramamohana Brahmāchari. After living and studying with his guru in a cave at the foot of Mount Kailas for seven and a half years, Krishnamacharya was sent back into the world to get married, raise children, and teach yoga.

As is the case with all great teachers, Krishnamacharya synthesized wisdom from various traditions and added his own genius, mixing the past and the present and pouring them into the future. In addition to *Patañjali's Yoga Sūtras*, he drew heavily from *tantrik* traditions in creating a system of yoga that has flourished around the world. And the synthesizing did not end with him. Today modern yoga teachers have access to vast amounts of information and ideas, some of which are rooted in ancient traditions, and some of which are recent inventions. The freedom that modern teachers have to create and recreate, to develop new ideas and test them, to mix and match and toss out what doesn't fit is unprecedented, especially as we are operating outside of the framework where yoga was originally born and crafted and refined over thousands of years. There are benefits to this freedom, and there are risks.

When we, as modern yoga teachers, call a modality or a class *yoga*, we are standing on thousands of years of tradition. We are carrying forward a torch lit by the first yogi, the Ādiyogi, Śiva Himself. A legend tells of how Matsyendranātha, a tenth century yogi, was thrown into a river by his parents just after his birth. He was swallowed by a fish, who swam to the bottom of the ocean where Śiva was teaching Parvati the secrets of yoga. Matsyendranātha listened carefully and began practicing according to what he heard, and after twelve years he emerged from the fish's belly as an illumined teacher.

This story personalizes a more ancient tale about Matsya the fish who, when Śiva caught him eavesdropping on his teaching to Parvati, named him Matsyendra, or Lord of the Fish, and told him to go and share what he had learned far and wide. And both stories emphasize that yoga is a secret teaching, shared intimately between the Ādiyogi Śiva and his beloved Śakti, and transmitted orally directly from teacher to student, with the line tracing straight back to Śiva himself. When new revelations emerged, they often sought legitimacy by claiming to come directly from Śiva as new additions, updates to the ancient canon based on the real issues of the day. Perhaps Śiva is still speaking, still intervening and inspiring us today, still bringing forth new revelations from the depth of His compassionate heart.

These stories also remind us that yoga is a precious gift to be treasured, a divine bestowal. Gratitude and humility are our best protection in this age of spiritual glamor. May we attend to our inner lives in a way that nurtures and cultivates these qualities, and so honor the exquisite gem that is Yoga. May we receive the infinite blessings that have poured from Śiva's Heart through time and space and into our modern lives. And may our practice be offered back and fulfill His compassionate intention to awaken all beings to their true nature as nothing but Śiva.

Chapter - 10

Savitri – A Legend And A Symbol

It's dinner time in Auroville in 2000, and I took my meal from the buffet and placed my plate on the wooden table. I sit down, swatting at the mosquitos beginning to gather around my exposed ankles. I close my eyes, breathe, and feel a surge of joy. An unexpected, sincere smile breaks out on my face. My nerves thrill with happiness and peace. I praise the goodness of the Divine Breath that has brought me to this place, this ecosystem that nourishes my soul in such a unique and exquisite way. I sing hymns of praise in my heart, open my eyes and let out an elated shout. This is my mealtime prayer, a moment of untamed gratitude born inside me in this land.

There is something special in the air, the water, the soil of Auroville, something planted there by the Mother, something given by Sri Aurobindo as a gift of his tapas. Just last year, as I was returning to Auroville from Kanchipuram, our car pulled off Koot Road, the highway that connects Puducherry and Tindivanam, and made a sharp turn to pass the Irumbai Śiva temple. We rounded the corner and saw the open fields that surround the temple, and I felt us enter a new ecosystem. I could feel what seems simplest to call the Mother's presence, her love embodied in the earth. It was a stark shift in atmosphere, and my heart softened and filled with the same joy and comfort that I'd first experienced almost in the same place twenty years before.

When the Mother returned by ship to Pondicherry after six years away, she described feeling Sri Aurobindo's presence a few miles from shore. She spoke of the radiance of the energy that they were bringing to the earth infusing Pondicherry and the surrounding area. This energy, this radiance, this spiritual light is also embodied in Sri Aurobindo's epic poem *Savitri*. The story is a revelation. It is profound, astonishing, exquisite language artfully woven. But beneath the form, the meter and the story, the poem breathes a certain divine fragrance into the being of the reader. It is a mantra that conveys the essence of its meaning directly, bypassing the mind and speaking straight to the inner being. I can do my best to give an overview, but only by reading it yourself can you catch a glimpse of what I mean.

History

Sri Aurobindo studied classical languages at King's College, Cambridge, at the end of the nineteenth century, and was widely considered one of the college's most brilliant graduates. He was deeply steeped in the ancient epics of the western world. And when he returned to India at the beginning of the twentieth century, he taught himself Sanskrit and began immersing in the spiritual texts of his native country. He was also a practitioner of yoga, experimenting intensely with various approaches that he found in the texts he read.

At some point in his yogic journey, Sri Aurobindo began writing an epic of his own, called *Savitri*. It appears that he started working on the poem in 1916, and a letter from 1931 states that the draft that existed at that point was found lacking, so he "started recasting the whole thing; only the best passages and lines of the old draft will remain, altered so as to fit into the new frame." He continued working on *Savitri* until his death in 1950, at which point his eyesight was so poor he could no longer write himself, and relied entirely on dictation. Nirodbharan, who served as his scribe during these years, wrote that he "would dictate line after line, and ask me to add selected lines and passages in their proper places...I wondered how he could go on dictating lines of poetry in this way, as if a tap had been turned on and the water flowed, not in a jet of course, but slowly...like a smooth and gentle stream." By the time of his passing, *Savitri* had reached over 23,800 lines, divided into twelve Books and forty-nine Cantos.

A Means of Ascension

Sri Aurobindo wrote that he "used *Savitri* as a means of ascension. I began with it on a certain mental level; each time I could reach a higher level I rewrote from that level...*Savitri* has not been regarded by me as a poem to be written and finished, but as a field of experimentation to see how far poetry could be written from one's own Yogic consciousness and how that could be made creative." Poetry as a form is supple and fluid. Metaphor and symbol can bring to life inner experiences and realities that are impossible to articulate in common language. Sri Aurobindo used the form to convey his own experiences and to deepen his own experiences as his immersion in yoga advanced.

This work is an incredible gift to the English language. All the other texts that I have described in this book were written in a language other than English, and for our English-speaking minds to understand them we need to translate. As I've mentioned, translation involves an inherent distortion of the text. We can try to retain and transmit as much of the spirit of the original as possible, but inevitably something is lost. That's why sometimes chanting mantras in Sanskrit, even if we don't understand their meaning, is more powerful than trying to dissect and interpret them.

That Savitri is written in English and directly articulates Sri Aurobindo's yogic experience provides us with unfiltered access to a yogic text that doesn't require translation. The mantra, the force of the words, pours through clearly, giving us the rhythm, the sound, and the meaning all wrapped together. To read it is a rare treasure for any yogic seeker whose primary language is English.

The Story of Savitri and Satyavan

The original story that he used as the base for *Savitri* comes from the *Mahābhārata*, the same epic that features the *Bhagavad Gītā*. In it, a great king named Aswapati prays for a son, and is granted a daughter by the Divine Mother in the form of Gāyatrī. The king names his daughter Sāvitrī, and she grows up to embody the wisdom, beauty, and grace of her divine origins. When it's time for her to get married, she travels around the land seeking a good match, and falls in love with the son of a deposed king named Satyavan.

When she comes back to tell her parents the good news, a sage tells them all that Satyavan is fated to die in one year's time. Sāvitrī decides that her love is stronger than this doom, marries Satyavan, and goes to live with him in the forest. On the day of his fate, Yama, the embodiment of death, comes to claim him. Sāvitrī argues with Yama, who is impressed with her intelligence, and grants her several boons. One boon that she chooses is to have a hundred sons. When Yama agrees, she reminds him that in order to have a hundred sons she will need to have her husband alive. Admitting defeat, Yama releases Satyavan to a joyful reunion with his beloved.

In the Author's Note at the beginning of his epic poem, Sri Aurobindo himself describes his version of the story:

The tale of Satyavan and Savitri is recited in the Mahabharata as a story of conjugal love conquering death. But this legend is, as shown by many features of the human tale, one of the many symbolic myths of the Vedic cycle. Satyavan is the soul carrying the divine truth of being within itself but descended into the grip of death and ignorance; Savitri is the Divine Word, daughter of the Sun, goddess of the supreme Truth who comes down and is born to save; Aswapati, the Lord of the Horse, her human father, is the Lord of Tapasya, the concentrated energy of spiritual endeavor that helps us to rise from the mortal to the immortal planes; Dyumatsena, Lord of the Shining Hosts, father of Satyavan, is the Divine Mind here fallen blind, losing its celestial kingdom of vision, and through that loss its kingdom of glory. Still this is not a mere allegory, the characters are not personified qualities, but incarnations or emanations of living and conscious Forces with whom we can enter into concrete touch and they take human bodies in order to help man and show him the way from his mortal state to a divine consciousness and immortal life.

Aswapati's Yoga

In *Savitri*, Sri Aurobindo has taken the frame of this ancient tale and reshaped it into a universal epic that traces the human aspiration for perfection that has characterized yoga for thousands of years. He begins with the Book of Beginnings, in which he provides an overview of the story. We begin in the stillness of the "hour before the gods awake", the symbol dawn that touches the emergence of light from darkness, movement from stillness, all creation from the empty vast. And we travel through the arc of Savitri's life until "the day when Satyavan must die." Sri Aurobindo plumbs the depths of wisdom and gathers the narrative of Aswapati's aspiration, and then brings us with him on what could only be a detailed and nuanced description of his own inner adventure.

In the original story, King Aswapati chanted the *gayatri mantra* incessantly for eighteen years. Sri Aurobindo invests fifteen cantos, a huge portion of the overall epic, in describing in radiant detail Aswapati's yogic journey through the many realms of creation.

"A Seer within who knows the ordered plan
Concealed behind our momentary steps,
Inspires our ascent to viewless heights
As once the abysmal leap to earth and life.
His call had reached the Traveller in Time.
Apart in an unfathomed loneliness,
He travelled in his mute and single strength

Bearing the burden of the world's desire.
A formless Stillness called, a nameless Light.
Above him was the white immobile Ray,
Around him the eternal Silences.
No term was fixed to the high-pitched attempt;
World after world disclosed its guarded powers,
Heaven after heaven its deep beatitudes,
But still the invisible Magnet drew his soul.
A figure sole on Nature's giant stair,
He mounted towards an indiscernible end
On the bare summit of created things."

We explore the realms where matter, life, and mind find their roots, and encounter the inhabitants and rulers of these kingdoms. And we climb toward the kingdoms of greater knowledge, where Aswapati's brain is

"...wrapped in overwhelming light,
An all-embracing knowledge seized his heart:
Thoughts rose in him no earthly mind can hold,
Mights played that never coursed through mortal nerves:
He scanned the secrets of the Overmind,
He bore the rapture of the Oversoul.
A borderer of the empire of the Sun,
Attuned to the supernal harmonies,

He linked creation to the Eternal's sphere.
His finite parts approached their absolutes,
His actions framed the movements of the Gods,
His will took up the reins of cosmic Force." (Book 2, Canto 15 p.302)

Aswapati finally arrives at the furthest reaches of manifestation, the edge of the knowable. In that silent expanse, where all words and thoughts and conceptions fail, he enters the emptiness that gives birth to form. And within that emptiness, he finds the Divine Mother. She appears to him, and his prayer is not for a son but for transformation and freedom from suffering for all humankind. He asks her to come and transform this aching earth, to "incarnate the white passion of thy force…let thy infinity in one body live…and with one gesture change all future time." She consents, saying that "one shall descend and break the iron Law, change Nature's doom by the lone spirit's power…Fate shall be changed by an unchanging will."

Birth, Quest, Love, and Fate

Savitri is born, and grows up "guarded in her spirit's luminous cell, alone mid men in her diviner kind. Even in her childish movement could be felt the nearness of a light still kept from earth, feelings that only eternity could share, thoughts natural and native to the gods." When she reaches the proper age, Aswapati sends her to seek her fortune and "venture through the deep world to find [her] mate." And amid her adventures she meets Satyavan, "the one for whom her heart had come so far."

His father Dyumatsena was a king, but when he became blind his brother sent him and his family to live in the forest. Satyavan explains that,

> "Outcast from empire of the outer light,
> Lost to the comradeship of seeing men,
> He sojourns in two solitudes, within
> And in the solemn rustle of the woods.
> Son of that king, I, Satyavan, have lived
> Contented, for not yet of thee aware,
> In my high-peopled loneliness of spirit
> And this huge vital murmur kin to me,
> Nursed by the vastness, pupil of solitude."

Savitri tells him that she must go home and share the joyful news of their love with her parents:

> "My heart will stay here in this forest verge
> And close to this thatched roof while I am far:
> Now of more wandering it has no need.
> But I must haste back to my father's house
> Which soon will lose one loved accustomed tread
> And listen in vain for a once cherished voice.
> For soon I shall return nor ever again
> Oneness must sever its recovered bliss
> Or fate sunder our lives while life is ours."

She returns home full of joy, "changed by the halo of her love," to find the sage Narad visiting with her parents. When she reveals the identity of her beloved, Narad is silent at first, but after being prompted by Aswapati and his queen, he speaks. "Twelve swift winged months are given to him and her: this day returning Satyavan must die."

Savitri's mother is bereft and quickly tries to convince her to leave Satyavan alone and find another partner. But Savitri will hear none of it. "My love shall outlast the world, doom falls from me helpless against my immortality. Fate's law may change, but not my spirit's will." Sri Aurobindo uses this opportunity for Narad to expound on the "Way of Fate and the Problem of Pain." The divine source of life hides from our eyes, and we are subject to the pain that has built this world:

> "Hidden in the mortal's heart the Eternal lives:
> He lives secret in the chamber of thy soul,
> A Light shines there nor pain nor grief can cross.
> A darkness stands between thyself and him,
> Thou canst not hear or feel the marvellous Guest,
> Thou canst not see the beatific sun...
> ...Pain ploughed the first hard ground of the world-drowse.
> By pain a spirit started from the clod,
> By pain Life stirred in the subliminal deep...
> ... The spirit is doomed to pain till man is free...
> ...The Great who came to save this suffering world
> And rescue out of Time's shadow and the Law,
> Must pass beneath the yoke of grief and pain;
> They are caught by the Wheel that they had hoped to break,
> On their shoulders they must bear man's load of fate...
> ... An exit is shown, a road of hard escape
> From the sorrow and the darkness and the chain;
> But how shall a few escaped release the world?
> The human mass lingers beneath the yoke.
> Escape, however high, redeems not life,
> Life that is left behind on a fallen earth."

But Savitri has come to help, to open a cosmic door and release us from the yoke of pain. Narad explains to the king and queen the special task that their daughter has taken on as the purpose of her embodiment. "Hard is the world-redeemer's heavy task." He encourages the queen to

> "Strive no more to change the secret will;
> Time's accidents are steps in its vast scheme...
> Sometimes one life is charged with earth's destiny,
> It cries not for succor from the time-bound powers.
> Alone she is equal to her mighty task...
> Her hour must come and none can intervene...
> Leave her to her mighty self and Fate."

So Savitri goes to live with her beloved, keeping from him and his parents the truth of his fate. She lives with this pain, this secret knowing. At first their shared life is blissful, but over time,

> "The more she plunged into love the anguish grew;
> Her deepest grief from sweetest gulfs arose.
> Remembrance was a poignant pang, she felt
> Each day a golden leaf torn cruelly out
> From her too slender book of joy and love."

She falls into a secret despair, dreaming "of her body robed in funeral flame," but aware that this would leave Satyavan's parents alone and helpless.

> One day, a "mighty Voice" comes and speaks to her:
> "Why camest thou to this dumb deathbound earth,
> This ignorant life beneath indifferent skies
> Tied like a sacrifice on the altar of Time,
> O spirit, O immortal energy,
> If 'twas to nurse grief in a helpless heart
> Or with hard tearless eyes await thy doom?
> Arise, O soul, and vanquish Time and Death...
> ...Remember why thou cam'st
> Find out thy soul, recover thy hid self,
> In silence seek God's meaning in thy depths."

Savitri's Yoga

Savitri embarks on an inner search for her soul, adventuring through similar terrain to that which her father traveled during his years of yoga. She encounters three manifestations of the Divine Mother, each with their own limitations. The first is the Mother of Sorrows, she who consoles all who suffer but has no power to stop the suffering.

The second manifestation is the Mother of Might, who has the power to face and vanquish darkness. Her description and voice are strikingly similar to that of Durga in the Devīmahatmya. She is powerful and fierce, but "The great obstinate world resists [her] Word. And the crookedness and evil in man's heart is stronger than Reason, profounder than the Pit...The cosmic suffering is too vast to heal."

And the third and final Mother is the "Madonna of light, Mother of joy and peace," who is "the mind of God's great ignorant world ascending to knowledge by the steps he made." She overcomes humanity's animal lusts and fear, the emotional tirades and visceral surges, but she cannot overcome doubt, and sees no reason for the spiritual quest. Savitri says to her:

> "Thou art a portion of my self put forth
> To raise the spirit to its forgotten heights
> And wake the soul by touches of the heavens.
> [Man's] hunger for the eternal thou must nurse
> And fill his yearning heart with heaven's fire
> And bring God down into his body and life.
> One day I will return, His hand in mine,
> And thou shalt see the face of the Absolute."

It is clear from these verses that Savitri has had some glimpse of who she is and why she lives. But the knowing is not fully embodied, integrated. The hour of purpose has not yet arrived. She leaves these Mothers with the promise of her return, and continues the quest for her soul, venturing deeper and deeper within until she discovers the "mystic cavern in the sacred hill…the dwelling place of her soul." Joined with her soul, she emerges from her meditation inspired with purpose and ready to face her fate. And in the course of her daily life with Satyavan, with "its small unchanging works and its spare outward body of routine," she continues her yoga, continues deepening her embodiment of the divine being that she is and preparing for the great work that she came to do.

She faces a being of intense evil that tries to frighten her from her path, and then receives comfort from a being of intense light who consoles her and encourages her to continue on. And she ventures on into the absolute stillness of nirvana. She touches the total absence from which the whole created universe arises, "the Truth where knowledge is not nor knower nor known." And she touches the total presence in whose heart that absence resides. She experiences herself as one with this embracing presence:

> "She was a single being, yet all things;
> The world was her spirit's wide circumference,
> The thoughts of others were her intimates,
> Their feelings close to her universal heart,
> Their bodies her many bodies kin to her;
> She was no more herself but all the world…
> Eternity looked out from her on time."

And then we arrive at the day of Satyavan's death. All that came before has been preparation for this holy moment. Sri Aurobindo revised most of *Savitri* before his own death, but he never got to this chapter. Some speculate that he could only write what he knew, and as he had not yet been through the process of death, he could not include it in the epic. Either way, what is included is a draft from an earlier version that describes Savitri, knowing the significance of the day, accompanying Satyavan on his errands in the forest. At some point while he's cutting wood he calls to her, falling down in agony, and asks her to hold him as he dies. She embraces him, and then feels the looming presence of death, "the Shadow of a remote uncaring god."

> This is the moment for which Savitri was born:
> "All in her mated with that mighty hour,
> As if the last remnant had been slain by Death
> Of the humanity that once was hers.
> Assuming a spiritual wide control,
> Making life's sea a mirror of heaven's sky,
> The young divinity in her earthly limbs
> Filled with celestial strength her mortal part.
> Over was the haunted pain, the rending fear:
> Her grief had passed away, her mind was still,
> Her heart beat quietly with a sovereign force."

The Book of Eternal Night

She stands and confronts Death, unwilling to let him take Satyavan away. Death commands her to stand down, and "pass lonely back to thy vain life on earth." He encourages her to let Satyavan go, explaining that by clinging to him she keeps him in suffering, while Death aims only to take him to "his soul death's calm and silent rest." Savitri releases her beloved, and Death leans down, lifts him, and carries him off. Savtiri follows. They pass through the realms between life and death, through a "strange hushed weird country" under "strange far skies," "a doubting space where dreaming objects lived." Eventually

Death stops and commands Savitri to turn back and "aspire not to accompany Death to his home, as if thy breath could live where Time must die." But:

> "The Woman answered not. Her high nude soul,
> Stripped of the girdle of mortality,
> Against fixed destiny and the grooves of law
> Stood up in its sheer will a primal force.
> Still like a statue on its pedestal,
> Lone in the silence and to vastness bared,
> Against midnight's dumb abysses piled in front
> A columned shaft of fire and light she rose."

Death continues on, and Savitri follows, "treading on the corpse of life, lost in a blindness of extinguished souls." Death speaks again, his stark, tragic logic crushing hope and aspiration and love:

> "What shall the ancient goddess give to thee
> Who helps thy heart-beats? Only she prolongs
> The nothing dreamed existence and delays
> With the labour of living thy eternal sleep.
> A fragile miracle of thinking clay,
> Armed with illusions walks the child of Time.
> To fill the void around he feels and dreads,
> The void he came from and to which he goes,
> He magnifies his self and names it God."

But he is impressed with the strength and courage that have carried her this far. So he offers her a boon:

> "Yet since thy strength deserves no trivial crown,
> Gifts I can give to soothe thy wounded life.
> The pacts which transient beings make with fate,

> And the wayside sweetness earth-bound hearts would pluck,
> These if thy will accepts make freely thine.
> Choose a life's hopes for thy deceiving prize."

Savitri replies undaunted:

> "I bow not to thee, O huge mask of death,
> Black lie of night to the cowed soul of man,
> Unreal, inescapable end of things,
> Thou grim jest played with the immortal spirit…
>
> …First I demand whatever Satyavan,
> My husband, waking in the forest's charm
> Out of his long pure childhood's lonely dreams,
> Desired and had not for his beautiful life.
> Give, if thou must, or, if thou canst, refuse."

Death assents, agreeing to give back to Satyavan's father Dyumatsena all that he had lost. He will receive his "kingdom and power and friends and greatness," though he mocks humanity's vain clinging to trifles like "pallid pomps" and the "sensuous solace of the light." And having agreed to Savitri's request, he commands her to turn back and go live out the rest of her days without Satyavan.

She again responds impervious to fear and despair:

> "World-spirit, I was thy equal spirit born.
> My will too is a law, my strength a god.
> I am immortal in my mortality.
> I tremble not before the immobile gaze
> Of the unchanging marble hierarchies
> That look with the stone eyes of Law and Fate.
> My soul can meet them with its living fire."

She demands that Death release her beloved, and if he won't she promises that "Wherever thou leadst his soul I shall pursue." The argument continues, with Death seeking to undermine Savitri's faith and love, "I, Death, am the one refuge of thy soul," and Savitri standing resolute:

> "O Death, who reasonest, I reason not,
> Reason that scans and breaks, but cannot build
> Or builds in vain because she doubts her work.
> I am, I love, I see, I act, I will."

The Debate of Love and Death

The Debate of Love and Death ensues, with Savitri answering each of Death's parries with unwavering love and wisdom. Death seeks to unburden her of her false hopes and pathetic ideals, and she reminds Death that though life is imperfect and fraught, it is also unfinished, and moving toward a perfection in which Death will be no longer needed. What awaits the earth and all her creatures is the embodiment of endless love, the perfect realization of truth, the seamless joining of spirit and matter. Not a vacant emptiness, but "a hidden Bliss is at the root of things." Everything in creation is made of joy, including evil, good, virtue and sin, "Its sap runs through the plant and flowers of Pain." All of evolution is a progressive emergence of this joy, a progressive enlightenment of all existence. And the hidden purpose of evolution will be fulfilled, the victory is assured.

> "Then is our being rescued from separateness;
> All is itself, all is new-felt in God:
> A Lover leaning from his cloister's door
> Gathers the whole world into his single breast.
> Then shall the business fail of Night and Death:
> When unity is won, when strife is lost

> And all is known and all is clasped by Love
> Who would turn back to ignorance and pain?
> "O Death, I have triumphed over thee within;
> I quiver no more with the assault of grief...
> ...My love eternal sits throned on God's calm;
> For Love must soar beyond the very heavens
> And find its secret sense ineffable;
> It must change its human ways to ways divine,
> Yet keep its sovereignty of earthly bliss.
> O Death, not for my heart's sweet poignancy
> Nor for my happy body's bliss alone
> I have claimed from thee the living Satyavan,
> But for his work and mine, our sacred charge.
> Our lives are God's messengers beneath the stars;
> To dwell under death's shadow they have come
> Tempting God's light to earth for the ignorant race,
> His love to fill the hollow in men's hearts,
> His bliss to heal the unhappiness of the world."

Even now Death resists

> "O priestess in Imagination's house...
> ... He who would turn to God, must leave the world;
> He who would live in the Spirit, must give up life;
> He who has met the Self, renounces self...
> ..In me all take refuge, for I, Death, am God."

And again and again Savitri demands that Satyavan be freed, allowed to take back up his body and his life, the life that Death deems a vain passage bound inevitably for its end in nought. Again and again Death denies, rejects, and uses reason to suck the sweetness and eloquence from her heart's speech.

> "Although he knew refusing still to know,
> Although he saw refusing still to see.
> Unshakable he stood claiming his right."

But finally:

> "A pressure of intolerable force
> Weighed on his unbowed head and stubborn breast;
> Light like a burning tongue licked up his thoughts,
> Light was a luminous torture in his heart,
> Light coursed, a splendid agony, through his nerves;
> His darkness muttered perishing in her blaze.
> Her mastering Word commanded every limb
> And left no room for his enormous will
> That seemed pushed out into some helpless space
> And could no more re-enter but left him void.
> He called to Night but she fell shuddering back,
> He called to Hell but sullenly it retired:
> He turned to the Inconscient for support,
> From which he was born, his vast sustaining self;
> It drew him back towards boundless vacancy
> As if by himself to swallow up himself:
> He called to his strength, but it refused his call.
> His body was eaten by light, his spirit devoured."

Savitri and Satyavan find themselves alone in the realm that had been Death's domain, but is now a radiant paradise. A divine voice welcomes them and praises their work, encouraging them to retire to Heaven and enjoy eternal sweetness. But Savitri knows that their work is still incomplete:

> "In vain thou temptst with solitary bliss
> Two spirits saved out of a suffering world;

> My soul and his indissolubly linked
> In the one task for which our lives were born,
> To raise the world to God in deathless Light,
> To bring God down to the world on earth we came,
> To change the earthly life to life divine."

The Divine Lord of Savitri's heart empowers and arms them with purpose, sending them back to earth to bring the light and truth and healing that they now embody. They return, illumined, full of promise and compassion, having chosen to forgo their own salvation and eternal freedom in order to uplift the earth.

> "With linked hands Satyavan and Savitri,
> Hearing a marriage march and nuptial hymn,
> Where waited them the many-voiced human world.
> Numberless the stars swam on their shadowy field
> Describing in the gloom the ways of light.
> Then while they skirted yet the southward verge,
> Lost in the halo of her musing brows
> Night, splendid with the moon dreaming in heaven
> In silver peace, possessed her luminous reign.
> She brooded through her stillness on a thought
> Deep-guarded by her mystic folds of light,
> And in her bosom nursed a greater dawn."

Sri Aurobindo's epic poem *Savitri* is a tale of sacrifice that carries the promise of universal liberation. Aswapati's human yearning for freedom is met by the Divine Mother's grace, and she agrees to embody upon the earth, to become fully human and face the human ordeal. As a human, Savitri longs and loves and hopes and fears. Her inner glow and embodied wisdom never fail, but at times she falters and doubts like every human.

Savitri's life is sacrifice, and the pain that she bears is her gift to all humanity. She traverses the horrors of Death's realm and faces his corrosive logic, she stands firm as his destroying wind buffets and seeks to blow her down. And in the end it is her love and knowing of herself that defeats Death and opens the door to "changing the earthly life to a life divine."

This is not just a story. It is the articulation of a truth that defies cynicism and factionalism. We stand today in the midst of a million insoluble problems converging upon each other. Our opposition to each other grows, we take sides and sling mud and hate and vitriol. There is no way out, no way through. The old ways must fall away, and something entirely new must emerge. Savitri is the divine assurance that we are not alone, that the Beloved is close, walking with us, as real and present as our human selves.

Savitri is an answer, a lamp to light the way, and its power comes not just from the substance but from the vibration. Reading the poem, silently and aloud, breathes the vibration into the world, introducing a healing medicine that can protect us in these times of travail. Savitri calls a luminous future to us, wraps us in a cloak of light, and shepherds us there. It is a cry, a trumpet, and a promise whispered to our aspiring hearts while our minds talk and sleep.

Bibliography

Below is a list of books that have inspired my writing. They are recommendations for further reading and also sources that I have drawn from as I wrote.

Chapters 1 and 2 – Rig Veda

Ghose, Aurobindo. *The Secret of the Veda*. Sri Aurobindo Ashram, 1982.

Ghose, Aurobindo. *Hymns to the Mystic Fire*. Sri Aurobindo Ashram, 1982.

Ghose, Aurobindo. Synthesis of Yoga. Sri Aurobindo Ashram, 1982.

Griffith, Ralph T.H. *The Rig Veda*. Digireads.com Publishing, 2013.

Julie of Light Omega. *From Light to Light: The Purification Process*. Light Omega Publishing, 2012.

Chapter 3 – Upanishads

Ghose, Aurobindo. *The Upanishads: Texts, Translations and Commentaries*. Sri Aurobindo Ashram, 1981.

Julie of Light Omega. *Living Yoga: The Practice of Embodiment*. Light Omega Publishing, 2012.

Chapter 4 – Rāmāyana

Menon, Ramesh. *The Ramayana: a Modern Retelling of the Great Indian Epic*. North Point Press/Farrar, Straus and Giroux, 2004.

Narayan, R.K. *Ramayana: A Shortened Modern Prose Version of the Indian Epic*. Penguin Classics, 2006.

Prasad, R.C. *Tulasidasa's Sri Ramacharitamanasa*. Motilal Banarsidass Publishers Pvt. Ltd., 2008.

Chapter 5 – Sankhya Kārikā

Bernard, Theos. *Hindu Philosophy*. The Philosophical Library, Inc, 1947.
Jha, Ganganatha. *An English Translation with the Sanskrit Text of the Tattva Kaumudi (Samkhya) of Vachaspati Mishra*. Bombay Theosophical Publication Fund, 1896.
Sharma, Dr. Har Dutt. *Iśvara Kṛṣṇa's Memorable Verses on Sāmkhya Philosophy, with the Commentary of Gaudapādācārya.*

Chapter 6 – Yogasūtra

Baba, Bengali. *The Patanjali Yogasutra with Vyasa Commentary*. N.R. Bhargawa, 1949.
Bachman, Nicholai. *The Yoga Sutras: An Essential Guide to the Heart of Yoga Philosophy*. Sounds True, Inc, 2010.
Satchidananda, Swami. *The Yoga Sutras of Patanjali*. Integral Yoga Publications, 2005.
Remski, Matthew. *Practice and All Is Coming: Abuse, Cult Dynamics, and Healing in Yoga and Beyond*. Embodied Wisdom Publishing, 2019.
Tigunait, Pandit Rajmani. *The Secret of the Yoga Sutra, Samadhi Pada*. Himalayan International Insitute of Yoga Science, 2018.
Tigunait, Pandit Rajmani. *The Secret of the Yoga Sutra, Sadhana Pada*. Himalayan International Insitute of Yoga Science, 2018.
White, David Gordon. *The Yoga Sutras of Patanjali: A Biography*. Princeton University Press, 2014.

Chapter 7 – Bhagavad Gītā

Bryant, Edwin F. *Bhakti Yoga: Tales and Teachings from the Bhāgavata Purana*, North Point Press, 2017.
Easwaran, Eknath. *The Bhagavad Gita*. Nilgiri Press, 2007.
Ghose, Aurobindo. Essays on the Gita. Sri Aurobindo Ashram, 1982.
Ghose, Aurobindo. *The Mahabharata: Essays and Translations*. Sri Aurobindo Ashram Trust, 1991.
Mitchell, Stephen. *The Bhagavad Gita: A New Translation*. Three Rivers Press, 2000.
Sargeant, Winthrop. *The Bhagavad Gītā*. State University of New York Press, 2009.

Chapter 8 – Devīmāhātmyam

Brown, C. Mackenzie. *The Song of the Goddess – The Devi Gita: Spiritual Counsel of the Great Goddess*, State University of New York Press, 2002.
Choudhary, Dr. Satya Prakash. The Glory of the Goddess - Devi Mahatmyam.
Janaswami, Ramakrishna. A Word for Word Meaning of Vak Suktam.
Kālī Devādatta. In Praise of the Goddess: *the Devimahatmya and Its Meaning*. Nicolas-Hays, 2004.
Menon, Ramesh. *Devi: The Devi Bhagavatam Retold*. Rupa Publications, 2006.
Sivananda, Swami. *The Devi Mahatmya*. The Divine Life Trust Society, 2017.

Chapter 9 – Tantrasāra and Thirumanthiram

Chakravarty, H.N. *Tantrasāra of Abhinavagupta*. Rudra Press, 2012.
Feuerstein, Georg. *Tantra: The Path of Ecstasy*. Shambhala Publications, 1998.
Hughes, John. *Hymns to Śiva: Utpaladeva's Śivastotravālī: Revealed By*

Swami Lakshmanjoo. Lakshmanjoo Academy, 2015.

Maharshi, Sri Ramana. *Arunachala Aksharamanamalai.*

Menon, Ramesh. *Siva: The Siva Purana Retold.* Rupa Publications, 2006.

Muller-Ortega, Paul Eduardo. *The Triadic Heart of Śiva: Kaula Tantricism of Abhinavagupta in the Non-Dual Shaivism of Kashmir.* State University of New York Press, 1989.

Muruganar, Muhavai Kanna. *Arunachala Aksharamanamalai.* Sri Ramanasramam, 2015.

Pope, G.U. *The Tiruvācakam: Sacred Utterances of the Tamil Poet, Saint and Sage Māṇikkavācagar.* University of Oxford, 1900.

Tirumular. *Tirumantiram.*

Wallis, Christopher D., and Ekabhumi Ellik. *Tantra Illuminated: the Philosophy, History and Practice of a Timeless Tradition.* Mattamayura Press, 2013.

Chapter 10 – Savitri

Ghose, Aurobindo. *Savitri.* Sri Aurobindo Ashram Trust, 1993.

Shraddhavan. *The English of Savitri, Volumes 1-4.* Savitri Bhavan, 2015.

Van Vrekhem, Georges. *The Mother: The Story of Her Life.* Rupa Publications, 2017.

General

Goldberg, Michelle. *Goddess Pose - the Audacious Life of Indra Devi, the Woman Who Helped Bring Yoga to the West.* Little, Brown Book Group, 2017.

Hixon, Lex. *Great Swan: Meetings with Ramakrishna.* Larson Publications, 2015.

Julie of Light Omega. *Teaching the Heart to Sing: A Guide to Shifting Consciousness at the Dawn of a New Age.* Light Omega Publishing, 1989.

Julie of Light Omega. *Living Unity: The Practice of Silence.* Light Omega

Publishing, 2012.

Kadetsky, Elizabeth. *First There Is a Mountain: a Yoga Romance*. Little, Brown and Company, 2004.

Mahony, William K. *Exquisite Love: Reflections on the Spiritual Life Based on Nārada's Bhakti Sūtra*. Sarvabhāva Press, 2014.

Sarma, Y. Subrahmanya. Narada's Aphorisms on Bhakti. Adhyatma Prakasha Press, 1938.

International Publications

Auroville Architecture
by Franz Fassbender

Auroville Form Style and Design
by Franz Fassbender

Landscapes and Gardens of Auroville
by Franz Fassbender

Inauguration of Auroville
by Franz Fassbender

Auroville in a Nutshell
by Tim Wrey

Death doesn't exist
The Mother on Death, Sri Aurobindo on Rebirth *Compiled by Franz Fassbender*

Divine Love
Compiled by Franz Fassbender

Five Dream
by Sri Aurobindo

Vision
Compiled by Franz Fassbender

Passage to More than India
by Dick Batstone

The Mother on Japan
Compiled by Franz Fassbender

Children of Change: A Spiritual Pilgrimage
by Amrit (Howard Shoji Iriyama)

Memories of Auroville - told by early Aurovilians
by Janet Feran

The Journeying Years
by Dianna Bowler

Auroville Reflected
by Bindu Mohanty

Finding the Psychic Being
by Loretta Shartsis

The Teachings of Flowers
The Life and Work of the Mother of the Sri Aurobindo Ashram *by Loretta Shartsis*

The Supramental Transformation
by Loretta Shartsis

The Mother's Yoga - 1956-1973 (English & French)
Vol. 1, 1956-1967 & Vol. 2, 1968-1973
by Loretta Shartsis

Antithesis of Yoga
by Jocelyn Janaka

Bougainvilleas PROTECTION
by Narad (Richard Eggenberger), Nilisha Mehta

Crossroad The New Humanity
by Paulette Hadnagy

Die Praxis Des Integralen Yoga
By M. P. Pandit

The Way of the Sunlit Path
William Sullivan

Wildlife great and small of India's Coromandel
by Tim Wrey

A New Education With A Soul
by Marguerite Smithwhite

Featured Titles

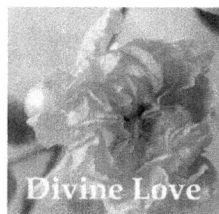

Divine Love

The texts presented in this book are selected from the Mother and Sri Aurobindo.
"Awakened to the meaning of my heart. That to feel love and oneness is to live. And this the magic of our golden change, is all the truth I know or seek, O sage."

Sri Aurobindo, Savitri, Book XII, Epilog

A Vision by the Mother

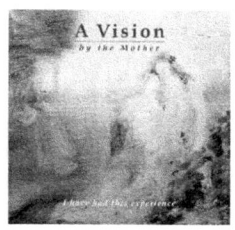

On 28th May 1958, the Mother recounted a vision she once had of a wonderful Being of Love and Consciousness, emanated from the Supreme Origin and projected directly into the Inconscient so that the creation would gradually awaken to the Supramental Consciousness. The Mother's account of this vision was brought out a first time in November 1906, in the Revue Cosmique, a monthly review published in Paris.

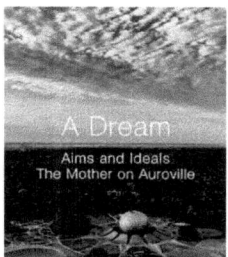

A Dream – Aims and Ideals of Auroville
the Mother on Auroville

50 years of Auroville from 28.02.1968 - 28.02.2018
Today, information about Auroville is abundant. Many people try to make meaning out of Auroville – about its conception, to what direction should we grow towards, and, what are we doing here?
But what was Mother's original Dream and what was her Vision for Auroville back then?

Matrimandir Talks by the Mother

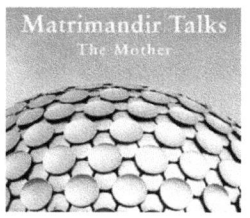

This book presents most of Mother's Matrimandir talks, including how she conceived the idea for this special concentration and meditation building in Auroville.

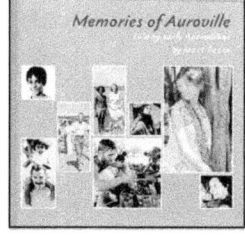

Memories of Auroville - Told by early Aurovilians

Memories of Auroville is a book about the very early days of Auroville based on interviews made in 1997 with Aurovilians who lived here between 1968 and 1973. The interviews presented in this book are part of a history program for newcomers that I had created with my friend, Philip Melville in 1997. The plan was to divide Auroville's history into different eras and then interview Aurovilians according to their area of knowledge. Our first section would cover the years from 1968 till 1973 when the Mother was still in her physical body.

The Way of the Sunlit Path

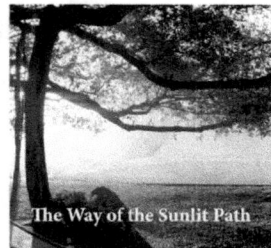

May The Way of the Sunlit Path be a convenient guide for activating this ancient truth as a support for a Conscious Evolution.
May it illumine the transformation offered to us in the Integral Yoga.

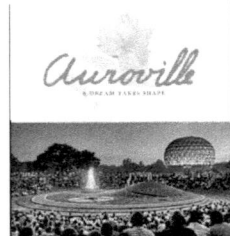

A Dream Takes Shape (in English, French, Hindi)

A comprehensive brochure on the international township of Auroville in, ranging from its Charter and "Why Auroville?" to the plan of the township, the central Matrimandir, the national pavilions and residences, to working groups, the economy, making visits, how to join, its relationship to the Sri Aurobindo Ashram, and its key role in the future of the world. This brochure endeavours to highlight how The Mother envisioned Auroville from its inception, some of the major achievements realised over the years, and some of the difficulties currently faced in implementing the guidelines which she gave.

Mother on Japan

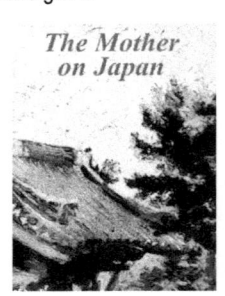

I had everything to learn in Japan. For four years, from an artistic point of view, I lived from wonder to wonder. And everything in this city, in this country, from beginning to end, gives you the impression of impermanence, of the unexpected, the exceptional... ...everything in this city, in this country, from beginning to end, gives you the impression of impermanence, of the unexpected, the exceptional. You always come to things you did not expect; you want to find them again and they are lost – they have made something else which is equally charming.

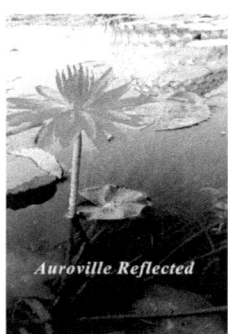

Auroville Reflected

On 28 February 1968, on an impoverished plateau on the Coromandel Coast of South India, about 4,000 people from around the world gathered for a most unusual inauguration. Handfuls of soil from the countries of the world were mixed together as a symbol of human unity. Why did Indira Gandhi, the erstwhile Prime Minister of India, support this development for "a city the earth needs?" Why did UNESCO endorse this project? Why does the Dalai Lama continue to be involved in the project? What led anthropologist Margaret Mead to insist that records must be kept of its progress? Why did both historian William Irwin Thompson and United Nations representative Robert Muller note that this social experiment may be a breakthrough for humanity even as critics commented, "it is an impossible dream"?

A House For the Third Millennium
Essays on Matrimandir

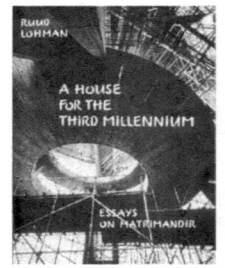

Nightwatch at the Matrimandir...
A cosmic spectacle; the black expanse above, the big black crater of Matrimandir's excavation carved deep into the soil. The four pillars - two of which are completed and the other two nearing completion - are four huge ships coming together from the four corners of the earth to meet at this pro propitious spot...

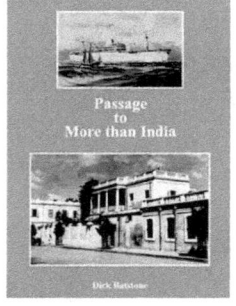

Passage to More than India

This book is a voyage of discovery. In 1959 the author, Dick Batstone, a classically educated bookseller in England, with a Christian background, comes across a life of the great Indian polymath Sri Aurobindo, though a series of apparently fortuitous circumstances. A meeting in Durham, England, leads him to a determination to get to the Sri Aurobindo Ashram in Pondicherry, a former French territory south of Madras.

Printed in the USA
CPSIA information can be obtained
at www.ICGtesting.com
LVHW021240071124
795952LV00014B/687